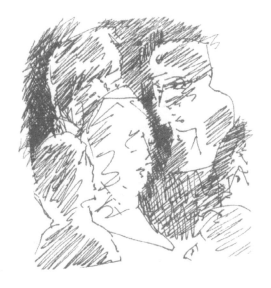

Illustration: 'Imagery in psychopathology' with kind permission of rogue-designs

MEMORY

Editors
Susan E. Gathercole and Martin A. Conway,
University of Durham, Department of Psychology, Science Laboratories,
South Road, Durham, DH1 3LE.
Tel: +44 (0)191 374 2625 Fax: + 44 (0)191 374 747
Email: S.E.Gathercole@durham.ac.uk

Aims and Scope of *Memory*

The Journal publishes high quality research in all areas of memory. This includes experimental studies of memory (including laboratory-based research, everyday memory studies and applied memory research), developmental, educational, neuropsychological, clinical and social research on memory. *Memory* therefore provides a unique venue for memory researchers to communicate their findings and ideas both to peers within their own research tradition in the study of memory and also to the wider range of research communities with direct interest in human memory.

Submission of manuscripts. Manuscripts should be prepared in APA format and submitted, in quadruplicate with a disk version, to Susan E. Gathercole and Martin A. Conway, Editors of *Memory*, University of Durham, Department of Psychology, Science Laboratories, South Road, Durham, DH1 3LE.

Memory is published by Psychology Press Ltd, a member of T&F Informa plc. Correspondence for the publisher should be addressed to the Head Office, 27 Church Road, Hove, East Sussex BN3 2FA, UK.

New subscriptions and changes of address should be sent to Psychology Press, Taylor & Francis Ltd, Rankine Road, Basingstoke, Hants RG24 8PR, UK. Please send change of address notices at least six weeks in advance, and include both old and new addresses.

US Postmaster: Please send address changes to pMEM, PO Box 1518, Champlain, NY 12919, USA.

Memory is available online: see *Psychology Online* at www.psypress.co.uk for information. Alternatively, please visit the journal website at http://www.tandf.co.uk/journals/pp/09658211.html

Memory is covered by the following abstracting, indexing and citation services: Biobase; Current Contents (ISI); Embase; Ergonomics Abstracts; Focus on Cognitive Psychology; LLBA; PsycINFO; Research Alert; SciSearch; Sociological Abstracts.

978-1-841-69967-7

Typeset by DP Photosetting, Aylesbury, Bucks

MEMORY, 2004, *12* (4), 387–388

A healthy imagination? Editorial for the special issue of *Memory*: Mental imagery and memory in psychopathology

Emily A. Holmes

MRC Cognition and Brain Sciences Unit, Cambridge, UK

Ann Hackmann

Oxford University, and Institute of Psychiatry, London, UK

Intrusive mental images in the form of flashbacks have long been recognised as a hallmark of post-traumatic stress disorder (PTSD). However, clinicians have become increasingly aware that distressing imagery is a more pervasive phenomenon. There appears to be a powerful link between imagery and autobiographical memory (Conway, Meares, & Standart, 2004 this issue). The field of autobiographical memory needs to account for disorders of remembering in psychopathology, including the reliving of past experiences in the form of imagery. While the role of mental imagery in psychopathology has been an under-researched topic, recently there has been a surge of interest.

This special issue of *Memory* on mental imagery and memory in psychopathology presents a novel series of papers investigating emotional, intrusive mental imagery across a wide range of psychological disorders. We include post-traumatic stress disorder, other anxiety disorders such as agoraphobia and social phobia, as well as psychosis, bipolar disorder, body dysmorphic disorder, and depression. The roles of imagery in symptom maintenance and in psychological treatment are explored.

Further studies using non-clinical samples address information processing issues and imagery qualities. These include innovative approaches to modelling cravings in substance misuse, and the role of imagery in conditioning aversions. Pioneering work is presented on vividness, emotionality, and the type of perspective taken in imagery. This special issue begins and ends with theoretical papers that provide complementary approaches; reviewing findings from a clinical psychology perspective and an autobiographical memory perspective.

New developments in cognitive therapy require a conceptual framework within which to understand imagery in specific psychopathologies. We believe that intrusive emotional imagery is not abnormal *per se* (e.g., Holmes, Brewin, & Hennessy, 2004), and seek to make links with accounts of "ordinary" processing. Conway's work on autobiographical memory may provide such a framework (Conway, 2001; Conway & Pleydell-Pearce, 2000). According to this model, images are thought to be forms of autobiographical memory, referred to as sensory perceptual knowledge that is experience-near. Indeed although they may be unaware at the time, patients often later report that images appear to be linked to autobiographical experiences. However, despite being a form of memory, images may

Correspondence should be sent to Emily Holmes, MRC Cognition and Brain Sciences Unit, 15 Chaucer Road, Cambridge CB2 2EF, UK. Email: emily.holmes@mrc-cbu.cam.ac.uk

Emily A. Holmes is at the MRC Cognition and Brain Sciences Unit, Cambridge, UK and also works as a Clinical Psychologist at the Traumatic Stress Clinic, London. Ann Hackmann is Consultant Clinical Psychologist at the Department of Psychiatry, Oxford University and the Institute of Psychiatry, London.

http://www.tandf.co.uk/journals/pp/09658211.html   DOI: 10.1080/09658210444000124

be experienced as actual events happening in the present, or as representing the imagined future, and projecting meaning for the self. Images may provide particularly potent means of carrying emotion and information about the self, compared to other forms of processing.

In this special issue of *Memory*, Conway presents novel insights that suggest imagery is highly associated with self-goals. Imagery can both reflect and maintain goals linked to psychopathology. An exciting consequence of this framework is that imagery may be used to resolve dysfunctional states in therapy. Imagery in psychopathology tends to be highly intrusive, distressing, and repetitive (Hackmann, 1998). It may arise "out of the blue", i.e., be directly triggered from autobiographical memory (Conway, 2001). Images can hijack attention and reflect negative self-goals.

Imagery may therefore understandably provoke a variety of cognitive and behavioural responses. For example, interpreting the image as representing fact rather than fiction, trying to block it out of mind, or avoiding triggers for the image. Cognitive behavioural therapy targets such responses because they are thought to maintain psychopathology in a vicious cycle. In contrast, responses that update the image in memory could break that cycle. Further, there is a role for positive, alternative images. Conway suggests that generating new images can generate new goals and thus ameliorate distress—an insight that may further enhance therapy.

We hope that this special issue of *Memory* will appeal to clinicians and experimental psychologists in the fields of memory and emotion. It provides a forum to forge links between experimental and clinical psychology. In bringing together a diverse range of research to the topic of mental imagery and memory in psychopathology, we hope this issue provides a unique opportunity to build on this exciting and rapidly expanding area.

REFERENCES

Conway, M. A. (2001). Sensory-perceptual episodic memory and its context: autobiographical memory. *Philosophical Transactions of the Royal Society of London Series B-Biological Sciences*, *356*(1413), 1375–1384.

Conway, M. A., Meares, K., & Standart, S. (2004). Images and goals. *Memory*, *12*, 525–531.

Conway, M. A., & Pleydell-Pearce, C. W. (2000). The construction of autobiographical memories in the self-memory system. *Psychological Review*, *107* (2), 261–288.

Hackmann, A. (1998). Working with images in clinical psychology. In A. S. Bellack & M. Hersen (Eds.), *Comprehensive Clinical Psychology*, *6*(14), 301–318.

Holmes, E. A., Brewin, C. R., & Hennessy, R. D. (2004). Trauma films, information processing, and intrusive memory development. *Journal of Experimental Psychology: General*, *133*, 3–22.

MEMORY, 2004, 12 (4), 389–402

Reflecting on imagery: A clinical perspective and overview of the special issue of *Memory* on mental imagery and memory in psychopathology

Ann Hackmann

Oxford University, and Institute of Psychiatry, London, UK

Emily A. Holmes

MRC Cognition and Brain Sciences Unit, Cambridge, UK

The authors provide an overview of the papers in the special issue of *Memory* on mental imagery and memory in psychopathology. The papers address emotional, intrusive mental imagery across a range of psychological disorders including post-traumatic stress disorder (PTSD), agoraphobia, body dysmorphic disorder, mood disorders, and psychosis. They include work on information processing issues including modelling cravings, conditioning, and aversions, as well as imagery qualities such as vividness and emotionality.

The overview aims to place the articles in a broader context and draw out some exciting implications of this novel work. It provides a clinical context to the recent growth in this area from a cognitive behavioural therapy (CBT) perspective. We begin with PTSD, and consider links to imagery in other disorders. The clinical implications stemming from this empirical work and from autobiographical memory theory are discussed. These include consideration of a variety of techniques for eliminating troublesome imagery, and creating healthy, realistic alternatives.

The significance of imagery in psychopathology is a highly promising area, as yet in its infancy. For example, cognitive therapy is a form of psychotherapy with an excellent evidence base, which involves explicitly identifying and modifying cognitions that maintain distress (Roth & Fonagy, 1996). A. T. Beck, the founder of cognitive therapy, emphasised that the therapeutic focus needs to be on *meanings*, which can be accessed through images, memories, and dreams as well as verbal thoughts (Beck, 1976). However, despite Beck's own interest in imagery, the major focus has been on verbal thoughts. The importance of imagery in psychopathology has perhaps still to be fully acknowledged, with notable exceptions, such as the seminal work of Lang and colleagues (see Lang, 1977). Despite this earlier work, links between the clinical and mainstream cognitive (experimental) psychology literatures in the area of imagery have not been fully integrated. For example, the mainstream cognitive literature does not appear to have associated mental imagery with emotion. This special issue of *Memory* also attempts to facilitate links between these two traditions.

Correspondence should be sent to Ann Hackmann, University Department of Psychiatry, Warneford Hospital, Oxford OX7 3JX, UK. Email: annhackmann@psych.ox.ac.uk

Ann Hackmann is a Consultant Clinical Psychologist at the Department of Psychiatry, Oxford University and the Institute of Psychiatry, London. Emily A. Holmes is at the MRC Cognition and Brain Sciences Unit, Cambridge, UK, and also works as a Clinical Psychologist at the Traumatic Stress Clinic, London.

We are extremely grateful to the contributors to this special issue for their contributing articles and inspiring feedback in this project.

---

http://www.tandf.co.uk/journals/pp/09658211.html   DOI: 10.1080/09658210444000133

There are several definitions of mental imagery, and that used in everyday language provides a useful starting point. The *Collins English Dictionary* (Harper Collins, 1995) defines an image as "A mental representation of something (especially a visual object) not by direct perception, but by memory or imagination". Thus defined, the term "imagery" encompasses memories and dreams as well as spontaneously triggered and deliberately self-generated images. The aims of this overview are as follows:

1. To summarise recent work on intrusive imagery in post-traumatic stress disorder (PTSD) and contemporary cognitive behavioural (CBT) models of PTSD.
2. To consider parallels between imagery in PTSD, the other anxiety disorders, and other types of psychopathology.
3. To discuss a range of studies that examine the nature and role of imagery more closely, highlighting the novel insights provided by the papers in this special issue and links to memory.
4. To cover new theoretical proposals about information processing, as well as experimental work on the qualities of mental imagery.
5. To consider the implications of these findings for developments in psychological therapy addressing imagery.

IMAGERY FOLLOWING TRAUMA

Perhaps the best place to start examining mental imagery, memory, and emotion is with intrusive imagery following trauma, since there is a clear autobiographical precipitant and the clinical phenomenology of trauma imagery is so striking. Re-experiencing the trauma, commonly as intrusive images, is a cardinal feature of post-traumatic stress disorder (PTSD) and acute stress disorder (ASD). We will summarise several properties of these intrusive, traumatic images—that is, that they: (a) are meaningful fragments of the trauma memory; (b) lack contextual information such as time and place; (c) are unintentionally retrieved; (d) encapsulate threatening meaning that may contradict later information; (e) contain themes of physical threat and threat to the sense of self.

Ehlers, Hackmann, and Michael (2004, this issue) summarise four recent studies. Ehlers, Hackmann, Steil, Clohessy, Wenninger, and

Winter (2002) found that a small number of intrusions (in any sensory modality) were experienced repeatedly. They often seemed to represent stimuli immediately preceding the first sign of danger, or just before a sudden shift for the worse in meaning. These features led Ehlers et al. (2002) to propose a "warning signal hypothesis" of intrusions in PTSD. It appears to accord well with the suggestion that some anxiety responses may be reactions to vivid, anticipatory images of conditioned stimuli (Mowrer, 1977). However, clinical observations suggest that a detailed model of human classical conditioning, incorporating the notion of stimulus revaluation (Dadds, Bovbjerg, Redd, & Cotmore, 1997: Dadds, Hawes, Smith, & Vaka, 2004 this issue; Davey, 1989) may be required to account for the complex phenomenology. For instance, the onset of PTSD symptoms can be delayed, with intrusive images and nightmares only appearing once the full significance of the traumatic event is appreciated. Someone raped on a date may be extremely upset, but not develop repetitive, intrusive imagery until she learns that her attacker raped and murdered another victim (Davey, de Jong, & Tallis, 1993; Ehlers et al., 2004 this issue).

Holmes, Grey, and Young (in press) note that while the majority of intrusions seem to be veridical fragments, a small number of images did not appear to be accurate representations of the index trauma. Such intrusions depicted fragments of an earlier trauma, or imagined events. The content of such images seemed heavily coloured by past experience.

Another feature of PTSD intrusions is that they appear to lack contextual information such as where and when the incident took place. The image seems to depict something happening here and now, rather than the past (Ehlers & Clark, 2000). It has also been suggested that trauma memories (unlike most other autobiographical memories) may occur without awareness that what is being experienced is actually input from memory. The memory lacks a "time code". It has been noted that as treatment unfolds, the images become less vivid and distressing, feel less "now", and their sensory qualities fade, until perhaps only a shadowy picture remains (Hackmann, Ehlers, Speckens, & Clark, in press). In a study of PTSD treatment by Hackmann et al. (in press), the patients reported that their intrusive images gradually decreased in frequency, and were *automatically triggered* less frequently, although the events could still be *deliberately* recalled. Hackmann et al. (in press) also observed that, given sufficiently strong cues, a "treated" trauma intrusion could still be automatically triggered.

An interesting, related feature of the treatment of PTSD imagery is the development of a "coherent narrative" during treatment (Foa, Molnar, & Cashman, 1995). Foa and colleagues noted that when the patients were asked to repeatedly describe their trauma, a more orga-nised narrative gradually emerged. The narrative changes could be assessed objectively using a lin-guistic coding system. Similarly, while studying naturally occurring changes in traumatic mem-ories, van der Kolk and Fisler (1995) found that initially patients were unable to put their mem-ories into words, and experienced them as somato-sensory images. Van der Kolk and Fisler asked the patients to describe the images they had experi-enced at various stages. They found that the images reached a peak of intensity at the point at which a coherent narrative began to emerge, and then following this they faded again. These find-ings suggest a shift from PTSD memories that involve intense, fragmented, now-like, imagery to memories that are less intense and more coherent, and that are grounded in a narrative context.

A further characteristic of intrusive images in PTSD is that they are often triggered unin-tentionally. A specific stimulus, present at the time of the trauma, may trigger the memory. For example, a patient experienced an intrusive memory of being attacked whenever she turned her head, but she could not explain why. It was later discovered that she had carried out this exact action immediately prior to her attack. When experienced in this way, the memories are typi-cally vivid, sensory experiences, accompanied by high affect, and the patient may not be aware of the trigger. These observations suggest that an *automatic* process may be responsible for retrieval of these memories. The moments in the trauma corresponding to the images may also be deliber-ately described with less affect, although attempts to describe them may sometimes spontaneously trigger affect-laden intrusions. Clinical experience suggests that intrusion-type images may also be deliberately self-generated, for example during the process of reliving/exposure therapy (Foa & Rothbaum, 1998). During reliving, the patient is asked to describe sensory and emotional aspects of the trauma in the first person, present tense. The resulting affect is initially very high, and the imagery vivid. Interestingly, small but important details of the trauma that have not previously

been recalled may suddenly appear to be remembered. These two different retrieval paths of trauma memories seen clinically map onto the distinction between "direct" (spontaneous) and "generative" (deliberate) retrieval in the model of autobiographical memory by Conway and col-leagues (Conway, 2001; Conway & Holmes, 2004; Conway; Meares, & Standart, 2004 this issue; Conway & Pleydell-Pearce, 2000).

Ehlers and Clark (2000) point out that in PTSD intrusions, the original emotions and sen-sations (i.e., those present at the time of trauma) can be persistently re-experienced with the origi-nal meaning, even if later information contradicts the original appraisal. It is as if knowledge in intrusions is not updated. In therapy therefore, one goal is to provide an update of the trauma memory, in a manner that incorporates the new information, such as using cognitive restructuring or image rescripting *during* reliving therapy (Ehlers, Clark, Hackmann, McManus, & Fennell, in press; Ehlers et al., 2003; Grey, Young, & Holmes, 2002). An interesting variant on this is provided by Conway et al. (2004 this volume). In one of their case studies the patient had a single flashback to the abuse, which conveyed dis-crepant meanings. In the image, the patient saw himself as he was now (an adult) rather than as a child, and the abuser was seen as a frail, old man (rather than a middle-aged man). This distorted image carried the meaning that he was a willing participant, and therefore guilty. This appraisal had never connected with the autobiographical knowledge that highlighted his vulnerability as a child at the time of the actual abuse. Interest-ingly, such information was partially present in the distorted image in terms of the feeling of his head against a radiator, which would be con-sistent with his short stature at the age of 6. Therapy made a bridge to integrate the two per-spectives via imagery transformation to a more realistic image, which reduced his guilt.

Holmes et al. (in press) asked people with PTSD to describe their intrusive images prior to treatment. Later, during reliving therapy in which they described the whole trauma, they were asked to report the "worst moments", known as "hot-spots". Intrusive images were found to correspond closely to the hotspots. In this and previous papers (Grey, Holmes, & Brewin, 2001; Grey et al., 2002) it was found that reported emotions associated with hotspots included fear, but also guilt, shame, disgust, sadness, and anger. This contrasts with the main focus of trauma researchers and clinicians to date, which has been on fear, helplessness, and horror, in line with diagnostic criteria (*Diagnostic and statistical manual of mental disorders,* 4th ed. DSM-IV; American Psychiatric Association, 1994).

Holmes et al. (in press) qualitatively analysed the cognitive themes reported in PTSD hotspots. Seven themes were identified, two involving threat to physical integrity (such as life threat), and five involving psychological threats to the sense of self (including abandonment, loss of esteem, loss of control, and future consequences). They found that themes associated with threat to physical integrity were less commonly reported than themes associated with psychological threat. Ehlers and Clark's (2000) model of PTSD highlights the observation that the threat can be physical, or may impact on the sense of self. For example, a patient may have an intrusion of a passer-by who seemed to ignore her during her attack, and re-experience cognitions and emotions associated with that hotspot, such as "he is not helping me", leaving her feeling helpless and angry. This could contribute to a sense of self as being "abandoned". It could be argued that intrusions provide an insight into people's "working self" associated with those moments in the trauma (cf. Conway & Holmes, 2004; Conway et al., 2004 this issue; Conway & Pleydell-Pearce, 2000). As such, intrusions can be seen as highly meaningful fragments of the trauma memory in terms of self.

CONTEMPORARY MODELS OF PTSD

Several models of PTSD have been reviewed in detail by Brewin and Holmes (2003a). They include emotional processing theory (Foa & Kozak, 1986; Rachman, 1980), a cognitive model of post-traumatic stress disorder (Ehlers & Clark, 2000), and dual representation theory (Brewin, 2001; Brewin, Dalgleish, & Joseph, 1996). Ehlers and Clark (2000) emphasise that there are two routes to the retrieval of autobiographical information about trauma: first, through higher-order meaning-based retrieval strategies and second, though direct triggering of images by associated stimuli. Personal events are normally incorporated into an autobiographical knowledge base that is organised by themes and personal time periods. Making connections and representations at the levels of themes and per-

sonal time periods is thought to enhance the first retrieval route and inhibit the second (Conway, 1997; Conway & Pleydell-Pearce, 2000). Ehlers and Clark (2000) propose that in persistent PTSD the trauma memory is poorly elaborated and inadequately integrated into its context with reference to time, place, and other autobiographical knowledge. This may explain the problematic intentional recall (weak semantic route to retrieval), and (in combination with strong perceptual priming for stimuli accompanying the traumatic event and strong associative learning) the easy triggering of images by internal and external stimuli.

Similarly, the dual representation theory of PTSD (Brewin, 2001; Brewin et al., 1996) proposes that during trauma two types of memory are laid down, one of which is deliberately and verbally accessible (VAMS), and the other more involuntarily accessible given situational cues (SAMS). SAMS are thought to involve sensory, physiological, and motor aspects of traumatic experience that support intrusions. VAMS are autobiographical memories that can be deliberately accessed and progressively edited, leading to the creation of memories encompassing the fact of having experienced the trauma, its context, etc. Detailed VAMS are thought to act to inhibit SAMS from intruding. Processes likely to be important in therapy include the creation of richer VAMS to inhibit SAMS from intruding, and incorporation of new knowledge into SAMS. To some extent these ideas parallel emotional processing theories (e.g., Foa & Kozak, 1986).

There is a tradition of dual process models in mainstream experimental psychology, which distinguish verbal and non-verbal memory information (e.g., Johnson, 1983; Paivio, 1986). Holmes, Brewin, and Hennessy (2004) argued that an area of overlap between the two main contemporary models of PTSD (Brewin et al., 1996; Ehlers & Clark, 2000) is the focus on broadly verbal versus sensory encoding processes at the time of a traumatic event, and the role of these in intrusive image recall. We also note that Conway's model of autobiographical memory (Conway & Pleydell-Pearce, 2000) also provides a complementary account of intrusive re-experiencing in PTSD. It is possible that such ideas about information encoding during stressful events, and subsequent intrusions, may have relevance in psychiatric disorders other than PTSD. If so, such findings might have important conceptual and therapeutic implications.

IMAGERY IN ANXIETY DISORDERS OTHER THAN PTSD

We suggest that there may be more similarities between the imagery in PTSD and imagery in other anxiety disorders than previously supposed. A number of studies have indicated that individuals with other anxiety disorders also have recurrent spontaneous imagery, which involves material in any modality (e.g., obsessive-compulsive disorder, de Silva, 1986; Speckens, 2003; health anxiety, Wells & Hackmann, 1993; social phobia, Hackmann, Clark, & McManus, 2000; spider anxiety, Pratt, Cooper, & Hackmann, in press; agoraphobia, Day, Holmes, & Hackmann, 2004 this issue). Such images are automatically triggered, and often appear to incorporate aspects of upsetting memories that carry important meanings. For example, Speckens (2003) reports that in obsessive-compulsive disorder one third of the intrusive images were reported to be *actual memories* of traumatic events, and two thirds of the other intrusive images also appeared to be closely linked to upsetting memories. As in PTSD, intrusions in other anxiety disorders can reflect events that occurred (or were imagined at the time), or can be formed following events the individual learned about from others. For example, some patients claim to have developed bird or spider phobias with intrusive imagery after watching well-known horror movies. People can also experience distressing intrusive images, which may not meet diagnostic criteria, following television broadcasts (Holmes, Creswell, & O'Connor, 2004).

It is also of interest that in generalised anxiety disorder, which is characterised by anxious and worrisome verbal thinking (rather than intrusive imagery) imagery is thought to play a crucial role. Pivotal work by Borkovec and colleagues suggests that verbal worry is used to inhibit aversive, negative imagery that might otherwise intrude (e.g., Borkovec & Inz, 1990; see also Nelson & Harvey, 2002).

Hackmann et al. (2000) studied the images of individuals with social phobia during anxiety-provoking situations. All reported recurrent, vivid, negative imagery of themselves, replicating Hackmann, Surawy, & Clark (1998). Images were typically of the self, viewed from an observer perspective (i.e., as if seen through the eyes of another person). All but one participant reported an upsetting memory (typically of criticism or bullying in adolescence), with which they

felt the current imagery was linked. These memories shared many sensory and meaning elements with the images.

There have been similar findings in agoraphobia. Day et al. (2004 this issue) report for the first time that patients with agoraphobia (which manifests for example, as a fear of leaving the house, being in crowds, etc.) reported experiencing repetitive, intrusive imagery in feared situations. In comparison, the non-clinical control group reported they did not experience imagery in these situations, although they were able to deliberately generate such images. When asked whether there was an experience associated with their recurrent image, all patients with agoraphobia reported a particular, distressing memory with similar content. The work of Conway and Pleydell-Pearce (2000) may aid our understanding of such results: the images appeared to be of extremely negative, self-defining moments when personal "goals" were severely challenged. The images were reported as being recalled involuntarily (Conway, 2001), which can "hijack" attention away from other current tasks. Experiencing intrusive images in agoraphobic situations could be very disruptive and influence ongoing behaviour, for example avoiding leaving the house. The way in which such negative images are interpreted by what Conway calls the "working self" could be destabilising. Clinically, this work has implications for our understanding of the onset and maintenance of agoraphobia, and the development of treatment strategies. It is suggested that imagery restructuring might be particularly useful.

Even if an intrusive image reflects a past episode, we emphasise that an anxious person may experience it as reflecting present or future danger. The patient may feel as if the image signals threat (cf. Martin & Williams, 1990), and act accordingly. This may be because such images lack contextual information, including a time code, as in PTSD. Anxiety images may feel very "believable". There may be an inability to appraise the image as "fantasy", rather than reality (cf. Holmes & Steel, 2004; Morrison, 2001). We believe that a key factor in the maintenance of several anxiety disorders may be the appraisal of intrusive imagery, followed by behaviour intended to reduce the perceived threat. Such behaviour may prevent updating of the original (negative) content of the image/memory and its meaning (Hackmann et al., 2000). A model of social phobia incorporating these elements to address specific imagery, has led to the development of an extremely effective treatment programme (Clark et al., 2003).

IMAGERY ACROSS PSYCHOLOGICAL DISORDERS OTHER THAN ANXIETY

In psychological disorders other than anxiety there may also be imagery associated with upsetting past events, accompanied by strong affect and behavioural reactions, and failure to update the images. Investigation of this has clear theoretical and practical importance, and this special issue of *Memory* charts several disorders in which imagery has not previously been extensively investigated. Osman, Cooper, Veale and Hackmann (2004 this issue) compared appearance-related imagery of patients with body dysmorphic disorder (BDD) to non-clinical controls. BDD is a clinically significant preoccupation with a perceived defect in appearance. Participants were asked to think about a recent time when they felt worried about their appearance, and whether they ever had visual images or other sensory impressions at such times. The BDD group reported images or impressions that were more negative, recurrent, vivid, and distorted than controls, and their images were typically viewed from an observer perspective. As in social phobia and agoraphobia, this BDD study also indicated links between images and troublesome early memories, such as being bullied or teased about appearance at school. These images may be problematic, if attention is focused on the distorted self-image rather than externally, where new information concerning the current reactions of others might be gathered. Such information could be used to update the image, and the meaning of the original, upsetting events. Therapy for BDD might usefully facilitate the formation of more realistic self-images.

In psychosis, images have also recently been proposed to be an important aspect of phenomenology (Morrison & Baker, 2000). Morrison, Beck, Glentworth, Dunn, Reid, and Larkin (2002) found that most patients experiencing psychotic symptoms such as hallucinations and delusions (diagnosed with schizophrenia, schizo-affective, or schizophreniform disorder) reported experiencing images in association with these psychotic symptoms. Many images were recurrent, and associated with high affect and upsetting memories. Morrison (2001) suggests that mental imagery is implicated in the maintenance of hallucinations and delusions, and supports the view that similar processes may be involved in anxiety and psychosis. He suggests that traumatic events may lead to some of the imagery observed in psychosis, and individuals may not be aware of the source of their images. Morrison suggests that in therapy, an analysis of the relationship between imagery and memories/perceptions of the real world may be beneficial. The key factor in the maintenance of images in psychosis may lie in their appraisal, rather than in the existence of the intrusions *per se* (i.e., the problem may be the fact that the images are experienced as reflecting reality, rather than being seen as images).

It is also possible that individuals with psychosis have particularly abundant imagery due to a longstanding proneness to intrusive imagery (Steel, Fowler, & Holmes, 2004). Steel et al. have argued that this may be because high schizotypy is associated with poor integration of contextual information during stressful events. In addition, there may be a failure to recognise triggers for images, and a failure to associate images with an index event. This could clearly cause distress, and contribute to the positive symptoms of psychosis.

Brewin and colleagues have investigated intrusive memories in depression (Brewin, Hunter, Carroll, & Tata, 1996; Kuyken & Brewin, 1994). They suggest that the frequency and other characteristics of intrusive memories in depression are remarkably similar to PTSD. Interestingly the thematic content of the intrusive memories in depression appeared to be similar to that of the more recent events that had triggered the current depression (e.g., relationship conflict and bereavement). In patients with cancer, people with higher levels of depression also had higher levels of intrusive memories than a group matched for cancer symptomatology but lower levels of depression. Events depicted in the intrusions included previous upsetting illness experiences of the self or others (Brewin, Watson, McCarthy, Hyman, & Dayson, 1998).

Mansell and Lam (2004 this issue) investigate autobiographical memory in remitted unipolar, and bipolar depression (also known as "manic depression"). Participants were asked to generate autobiographical memories in response to positive and negative cue words. Consistent with the above findings, certain themes were particularly evident and included patients' memories of past depressive episodes, and of being told they were a failure. The memories were also classified as specific or general. Models of autobiographical memory (e.g., Conway & Pleydell-Pearce, 2000) suggest that memory is organised hierarchically, with upper layers containing general information, while the lowest layer contains "event-specific knowledge" (ESK). The tendency to recall general rather than specific memories has been shown to be characteristic of certain psychological disorders, such as depression (Williams & Scott, 1988) and PTSD (McNally, Lasko, Macklin, & Pitman, 1995). Overgeneral memory bias has been shown to be associated with poor problem-solving ability (Scott, Stanton, Garland, & Ferrier, 2000), which may be a maintenance factor. Mansell and Lam (2004 this issue) found that relative to the remitted unipolar group, the remitted bipolar group reported more general than specific memories, and more recollections of the negative memories in everyday life. The study also revealed that across the sample, almost all specific memories involved mental imagery, while only approximately half the general memories did so. These findings suggest that specific memories may be particularly associated with imagery, a finding consistent with an earlier non-clinical study by Williams, Healy, and Ellis (1999). Precise relationships between over general memory bias and intrusive memories remain to be explored.

INFORMATION PROCESSING AND QUALITIES OF MENTAL IMAGERY

This special issue of *Memory* also covers groundbreaking work in non-clinical samples, investigating information processing and the qualities of mental imagery and memory with respect to emotion. Insights from psychopathology can fuel such research areas. Intrusive, emotional memory is a little understood topic in the mainstream memory arena. One contemporary viewpoint is that various facets of information processing (such as imagery) exist on continua throughout the population from non-psychopathological to psychopathological processing (cf. Harvey, Watkins, Mansell, & Shafran, in press). It can therefore be informative to investigate processes in analogue populations as well as conducting research in clinical populations (Holmes, in press). Our knowledge of how intrusive images arise in response to processing during encoding of a traumatic event cannot be ethically investigated during real trauma, but can be studied in the

laboratory using the stressful film paradigm (Holmes, Brewin, & Hennessy, 2004).

Experimental work can also help tease out various predisposing factors in the development of distressing imagery. For example, Holmes and Steel (2004) used the stressful film paradigm in a student population, and found that individuals with high scores on a measure of schizotypy reported significantly more intrusive memories than those with low scores. Schizotypy is a construct used to describe the tendency to experience psychotic-like symptoms, lying on a continuum throughout the population. However, there are likely to be multiple reasons why some people may experience more intrusive images than others. Overall, analogue methodology provides a tool to probe questions such as intrusion development, and how images may play a role in the acquisition and maintenance of psychological dysfunctions.

One role that images may play is that of representing desired outcomes. May, Andrade, Panabokke and Kavanagh (2004 this issue) have been pursuing important new work in the area of substance misuse and craving. They have taken a cognitive model from experimental psychology known as Interacting Cognitive Subsystems or ICS (Barnard & Teasdale, 1991) and have used this to make predictions about what happens when someone experiences a craving for a substance. It should be noted that the work by Teasdale and colleagues (e.g., Teasdale, 1999) has important implications for imagery beyond substance misuse, a discussion of which is unfortunately beyond the scope of this article. Substance misuse is notoriously difficult to treat, and thus provides an example of where ideas from experimental psychology may be called in to assist. The approach by May et al. (2004 this issue) exemplifies the utility of developing our understanding in a clinical area using work from mainstream psychology. This recent work has attracted considerable interest (Baker, 2003; Connor, 2003; May, 2003).

May et al. (2004 this issue) compare two theories of clinical cravings using the ICS perspective. Accordingly, they argue that their own model, the Elaborated Intrusions theory of craving, may provide the most useful approach. Their theory proposes that mental imagery is central to craving. That is, in response to triggers, people experience images of a substance, such as a cigarette. This intrusive image is initially associated with positive affect and therefore elaborated, fuelling the subjective experience of craving and realisation of substance deficit. This process disrupts other ongoing cognitive activities. The authors present data on the subjective experience of everyday desires in a large non-clinical sample. The results support the view that cravings are experienced as arriving spontaneously, involve mental imagery in a variety of modalities, and initially lead to pleasurable anticipation. This approach allows cognitive processing in craving to be dissected into component parts. From a clinical perspective, it certainly points to the utility of targeting intrusive images of craved substances as part of psychological therapy.

The opposite of craving a substance is having an aversion to it. In aversions, a role that imagery may play is to promote a negative reaction and avoidance, perhaps similarly to images in anxiety as discussed earlier. Dadds et al. (2004 this issue) investigated individual differences in imagery ability and the tendency to report specific aversions, for example to certain foods. Participants were given questionnaire measures of imagery ability, absorption in events or imagery, neuroticism, and disgust proneness. In addition, they completed a checklist of specific aversions including food, people, and places, and superstitious avoidance behaviour. Results indicated that a high level of imagery ability was associated with a high level of aversions, even after controlling for neuroticism and proneness to disgust. The authors discuss their theory that more vivid imagery might enhance aversive learning. This is based on principles of conditioning—that is, a mental image can have a similar function to a real stimulus in learning to associate innocuous stimuli with threatening, biologically relevant outcomes. This idea provides another insight into why images may be effective in evoking and maintaining negative emotion in psychopathology.

"Vividness" is a cornerstone topic in the study of mental imagery, but surprisingly little research has investigated vividness of mental imagery in relation to emotion. Drawing from clinical work in depression and PTSD, Bywaters, Andrade and Turpin (2004a, 2004b this issue) present two papers studying intrusive memories in a nonclinical sample. In the first, they studied the vividness, valence, and frequency of intrusive images of autobiographical memories. Participants reported experiencing unpleasant, but more frequently pleasant, intrusive memories in everyday life. Deliberately formed images of intrusive memories were reported to be more vivid than deliberately formed images of non-intrusive memories, regardless of valence or arousal. Interestingly, the authors also provide data on psychophysiological responses to imagery. This work supports other claims that intrusive memories are a feature of "normal" memory, not a sign in themselves of psychopathology.

In their second study, Bywaters and colleagues probed memory not of autobiographical events, but for picture stimuli. Their focus was the determinants of the vividness of visual imagery for such material. The more extremely valenced and arousing pictures were associated with more vivid imagery. However, as the interval increased between viewing a picture and forming an image of it, the contribution of these stimulus variables declined somewhat and that of individual differences (e.g., BDI score) increased. One striking finding was that after 1 year, some participants reported still experiencing intrusive imagery of some negative picture material. This may have ethical implications for research in this area, which perhaps may best be conducted in the context of researchers with clinical experience. Such studies underscore the perspective that the vivid, negative, intrusive imagery seen in patient populations also occurs, albeit it in a less extreme form, in non-clinical populations. If more emotional autobiographical memories are more vivid, it remains to be explored how this has an impact in psychopathology. For example, highly vivid images may be more compelling and believable than less vivid ones. It would be helpful if theories of autobiographical memory furthered our understanding of what determines imagery intrusiveness and vividness.

Other findings support the view that imagery vividness is not simply a function of trait differences, but is also affected by the individual's particular concerns. For example, Pratt et al. (in press) found that self-generated and spontaneous images of spiders in individuals with high spider anxiety were more vivid and distressing than in those with low spider anxiety. In contrast, self-generated images of butterflies did not differ in any of their characteristics in the spider anxious and the control groups.

Stopa and Bryant (2004 this issue) aimed to investigate Libby and Eibach's (2002) hypothesis that individuals are more likely to use the observer perspective when recalling memories of social situations that are incongruent with current self-concept. Limited support was found for this: high socially anxious (non-clinical) participants were more likely to recall the second of two self-incongruent memories from an observer perspective, but no more likely than low socially anxious people to recall self-congruent memories from this perspective. Furthermore, a measure of trait public self-consciousness was related to imagery vividness. This exploratory study provides a stepping-stone for future research that is likely to be highly relevant to psychopathology. Clinicians are familiar with patients reporting out-of-body experiences and images, and it can be difficult to help patients with their distress associated with these. Taking an observer perspective, at time when an individual has discrepancies in self-concept, may serve a possible protective function (cf. Conway et al., 2004 this issue). Working directly on issues of the self and potential discrepancies may therefore be a useful focus of therapy.

THERAPEUTIC EFFECTS OF MANIPULATING IMAGERY

Clinical practice would benefit from a body of information concerning the effects of manipulating imagery (Hackmann, 1998). Hirsch, Meynen, and Clark (2004 this issue) investigated individuals with high social anxiety. Their paper elegantly demonstrates the power of self-generated negative imagery to adversely affect behaviour, increase distress, and inadvertently contaminate the social situation. In contrast, self-generated imagery of being relaxed in a social situation had immediate beneficial effects. This study suggests that spontaneously occurring negative self-images may be causal in the maintenance of social phobia. As stated earlier, it has been suggested that in social phobia, negative images are based on previous distressing experiences. Further, safety behaviours (i.e., behaviours an individual engages in to try to keep themself safe), including avoidance, may lead to a failure to update the images (Hackmann et al., 2000). Hirsch et al.'s paper has important implications for therapy. Merely summoning up a non-negative image of the self led to less anxiety and better performance in the eyes of other people.

There may be several techniques for working with images. In PTSD images are traditionally worked through by encouraging the patient to relive them, access the meanings, and challenge distorted appraisals. In social phobia, Hirsch et al.'s research suggests that less negative images could be "substituted" for more negative ones. It is conceivable that with higher levels of social

anxiety and chronicity this could be more difficult, since autobiographical memories of being relaxed in social situations might be harder to access. However, earlier work by Hirsch et al. (Hirsch, Clark, Mathews, & Williams, 2003) demonstrated that even individuals with social phobia benefited a great deal from holding a non-negative image in mind. It is also possible that, while image substitution may provide temporary relief, lasting improvement may require more work on the original upsetting memories.

Gilbert and Irons (2004 this issue) provide an exploratory study, again involving active manipulation of imagery. As these authors point out, shame and self-criticism underpin many features of depression, anxiety, and other disorders, and the early origins for self-criticism may lie in emotional memories of being criticised. These authors hypothesise that self-critics may have underdeveloped processing systems for generating supportive and compassionate self-evaluations. Their study uses a self-report diary to capture key qualities of self-criticism, and to explore participants' experience of attempting to generate, on a regular basis, compassionate imagery for the self. Participants were drawn from a self-help group for chronic depression who agreed to monitor their thoughts over a number of weeks. Participants provided a number of novel insights into the power of self-criticism, and the complexity and difficulties of trying to be more compassionate to self. Indeed, one participant found the effort distressing, as her effort to generate a compassionate image often turned into the memory of an abusive ex-husband. As these authors point out, compassionate imagery has been used for thousands of years as a healing process (e.g., in Buddhism), but there is much we have yet to understand about the forms, functions, and value of compassionate imagery in alleviating self-criticism and other psychological difficulties.

In this special issue of *Memory*, Morrison (2004 this issue) presents a single case study illustrating the clinical applications of his cutting edge work on cognitive behaviour therapy (CBT) for psychosis. As previously mentioned, some people with psychosis (who may be diagnosed with schizophrenia, schizo-affective disorder. or delusional disorder) have symptoms in the form of intrusive, distressing imagery associated with their hallucinations and delusions. In this study, the key therapeutic technique used to work with such negative imagery was at a "metacognitive" level, i.e., reflecting on the patient's appraisal of the image and their response to it. Challenging the validity of appraisals of images associated with the patient's persecutory delusions reduced his distress and conviction in relation to these beliefs. In addition, verbal challenging of their validity was enhanced by the use of imagery techniques, which pressed home the message that the images were "only images", and could be manipulated. This paper well illustrates the usefulness of single case design methodology in testing novel treatment approaches. In the rapidly developing new area of CBT for psychosis, the use of imagery techniques seems a promising way forward.

We note that there are several therapeutic tools for working with distressing mental imagery in psychopathology. As two of the above-mentioned, treatment-related papers in this special issue indicate, one idea is what we have called "image substitution". It should be noted that this is very recent work, and that in CBT there is a stronger tradition of working with imagery in ways that involve examining the meanings of the image and finding alternatives, rather than swapping it. For example, in the anxiety disorders, a patient can be helped to test the assumption that images reflect reality using verbal discussion techniques combined with what is known clinically as a "behavioural experiment". In a behavioural experiment the patient makes predictions of what might happen in a given anxiety-provoking situation, operationalising their predictions very clearly (Bennett-Levy et al., 2004). They are then encouraged to enter the situation, take careful note of what happens, and compare the outcome with their predictions, expressed in words and/or images. For example, a patient might be asked to carefully process video feedback of a conversation during which they blushed, and consider whether they actually looked as red as they imagined (Harvey, Clark, Ehlers, & Rapee, 2000). Video feedback might provide convincing new images for image substitution.

Another technique is to engage in fuller emotional processing and contextualisation of the image. This idea fits well with Conway and Pleydell-Pearce's (2000) ideas about integrating intrusive, event-specific knowledge (images) into the autobiographical memory system. PTSD models (e.g., Brewin et al., 1996a; Ehlers & Clark, 2000) suggest that traumatic memories need to be accessed in rich sensory detail. One way that reliving / exposure therapy is believed to function is via conditioning principles such as extinction learning. While distressing, exposure therapy also appears to help the patient begin to organise the memory, and link it to other autobiographical knowledge, so that it is seen as a single event without implications for the present and the future. There may also be a role for drawing in ideas from the working memory literature, to facilitate exposure (Andrade, Kavanagh, & Baddeley, 1997).

More recently, clinical work on hotspots in trauma (cf. Grey et al., 2002; Holmes et al., 2004) suggests that re-experiencing symptoms in PTSD may be treated, not by focusing on the entire trauma memory, but by just focusing on troublesome aspects that intrude as images (i.e., hotspots). In such work, the contents of the image are clearly identified, the negative meaning for self discussed, and a positive update or alternative for self integrated with that moment. This can be done both verbally and by constructing a positive image designed to convey the new meaning.

We are also inspired by findings from the experimental literature that contribute to therapy development using imagery. One example comes from Kavanagh, Freese, Andrade, and May (2001). They used an analogue treatment trial to investigate the utility of using concurrent tasks to reduce the distress caused by emotional imagery. Secondary tasks may disrupt emotional imagery by loading on visuospatial working memory (Baddeley & Andrade, 2000). These initial results indicated that a visuo-spatial task initially reduced vividness and distress, but this was not maintained at a 1-week follow-up. However, it may still be extremely useful to have a therapeutic tool that could at least initially reduce emotionality, as this may facilitate a patient's willingness to engage in emotional, distressing imagery in therapy. A concurrent task could provide extra steps in "stepwise" exposure treatments for PTSD and other anxiety disorders. There is some preliminary evidence that disrupting visual imagery may reduce cravings for cigarettes in deprived smokers (Panabokke, May, Eade, Andrade, & Kavanagh, 2004).

It remains to be seen whether the use of imagery techniques such as fuller emotional processing and contextualisation of images would be efficacious in disorders other than PTSD. We suggest that the appraisal of automatically triggered imagery appears to be an important common maintenance factor across psychological disorders. Distorted appraisals trigger distress and/or maladaptive behaviour, which can block the updating and contextualisation of recurrent imagery. Cognitive therapy aims to modify these appraisals, leading the automatically triggered images to subside (for a broader discussion on this issue, see Mansell, 2000). We believe it is likely that targeting particular memories that appear linked to current distressing imagery in the other anxiety disorders, body image disorders, mood disorders, psychosis and so forth, may also be effective. We have also noted that there are several additional techniques for working with imagery, including using metacognitive strategies. For a review of methods of working with images in therapy see Hackmann (1998).

In addition to attempting to "demolish" outdated negative imagery, there may also be a role for using procedures that enable patients to access more positive memories and images, as well as construct positive futures for themselves. In other disorders, such as craving in substance misuse, the unfortunate role of "positive" imagery needs to be tackled. However, we believe that strategies for treating problematic imagery that induces craving, may be similar in principle to treating imagery that induces anxiety and aversions. In the development of therapeutic techniques using imagery, the role of the self and identity (Conway & Pleydell-Pearce, 2000) is also likely to be pivotal.

CONCLUSIONS AND LINKS WITH AUTOBIOGRAPHICAL MEMORY

If imagery in psychotherapy has been under-researched, this special issue of *Memory* has provided a unique opportunity for researchers and clinicians to pool recent observations. The body of papers presents novel findings suggesting that imagery is widespread in psychopathology, rather than being restricted to PTSD. This special issue charts imagery prevalence in a further range of disorders including agoraphobia, body dysmorphic disorder, and bipolar disorder. We also present new findings on the role of imagery in disorders of imagery processing, such as cravings and aversions. Studies in non-clinical samples usefully explore qualities of emotional imagery, such as vividness and perspective. Finally, the special issue turns to the use of imagery in therapy, and we present recent novel suggestions against a backdrop of existing therapeutic techniques addressing problematic imagery. Connecting ideas about mental imagery and psychopathology to the area of autobiographical memory forges links of both theoretical and clinical significance. We believe that this connection should be used to generate future directions for theory-driven clinical innovation (Salkovskis, 2002).

The last paper in the series in this special issue of *Memory*, by Conway et al. (2004 this issue) brings together the previous papers from an autobiographical memory perspective. It also presents a fresh development of his theory (Conway, 2001; Conway & Pleydell-Pearce, 2000) by considering in more detail the roles of mental imagery in autobiographical memory, and specifically in psychopathology. From a clinical psychology perspective, developing the clinical relevance of this theory has several exciting implications. It highlights the strong links between images and goals for an individual, for example that images reflect moments when goals are threatened. It has several clinical implications in terms of how to break the cycle of negative, distressing imagery. Since images are the "language" of the goal system, creating images in therapy that represent more positive goals could be one way of "speaking" to that persons' goal system. Specifically targeted, positive imagery could help someone update their goals associated with ongoing psychopathology. This is an area that demands future exploration in clinical research and practice.

REFERENCES

American Psychiatric Association (1994). *The diagnostic and statistical manual for mental disorders* (4th ed.). Washington, DC: American Psychiatric Association.

Andrade, J., Kavanagh, D., & Baddeley, A. (1997). Eye-movements and visual imagery: A working memory approach to the treatment of post-traumatic stress disorder. *British Journal of Clinical Psychology*, *36*, 209–223.

Baddeley, A. D., & Andrade, J. (2000). Working memory and the vividness of imagery. *Journal of Experimental Psychology-General*, *129*(1), 126–145.

Baker, J. (2003). Flickering chequerboard curbs smokers' cravings. *Nature Science Update*. Retrieved 28 November 2003, from http://www.nature.com/nsu/030908/030908-18.html

Barnard, P. J., & Teasdale, J. D. (1991). Interacting cognitive subsystems: A systemic approach to cognitive-affective interaction and change. *Cognition and Emotion*, *5*, 1–39.

Beck, A. T. (1976). *Cognitive therapy and the emotional disorders*. New York: International Universities Press.

Bennett-Levy, J., Butler, G., Fennell, M. J. V., Hackmann, A., Mueller, M., & Westbrook, D. (in press).

The Oxford guide to behavioural experiments in cognitive therapy. Oxford: Oxford University Press.

Borkovec, T. D., & Inz, J. (1990). The nature of worry in generalized anxiety disorder: A predominance of thought activity. *Behaviour Research and Therapy, 28*(2), 153–158.

Brewin, C. R. (2001). A cognitive neuroscience account of posttraumatic stress disorder and its treatment. *Behaviour Research and Therapy, 39*(4), 373–393.

Brewin, C. R., Dalgleish, T., & Joseph, S. (1996a). A dual representation theory of posttraumatic stress disorder. *Psychology Review, 103*(4), 670–686.

Brewin, C. R., & Holmes, E. A. (2003a). Psychological theories of posttraumatic stress disorder. *Clinical Psychology Review, 23*(3), 339–376.

Brewin, C. R., & Holmes, E. A. (2003b). Psychology and cognitive processing in PTSD. *Psychiatry, 2*(6), 28–31.

Brewin, C. R., Hunter, E., Carroll, F., & Tata, P. (1996b). Intrusive memories in depression: An index of schema activation? *Psychological Medicine, 26*(6), 1271–1276.

Brewin, C. R., Watson, M., McCarthy, S., Hyman, P., & Dayson, D. (1998). Intrusive memories and depression in cancer patients. *Behaviour Research and Therapy, 36*(12), 1131–1142.

Bywaters, M., Andrade, J., & Turpin, G. (2004a). Determinants of the vividness of visual imagery: The effects of delayed recall, stimulus affect and individual differences. *Memory, 12*, 467–478.

Bywaters, M., Andrade, J., & Turpin, G. (2004b). Intrusive and non-intrusive memories in a non-clinical sample. *Memory, 12*, 479–488.

Clark, D. M., Ehlers, A., McManus, F., Hackmann, A., Fennell, M., Campbell, H. et al. (2003). Cognitive therapy versus fluoxetine in generalized social phobia: A randomized placebo-controlled trial. *Journal of Consulting and Clinical Psychology, 71*, 1058–1067.

Connor, S. (2003, September 12). Why smokers could be programmed to kick habit. *The Independent.*

Conway M. A. (1997). Past and present: Recovered and false memories. In M. A. Conway (Ed.), *Recovered and false memories* (pp. 150–191) Oxford: Oxford University Press.

Conway, M. A. (2001). Sensory-perceptual episodic memory and its context: Autobiographical memory. *Philosophical Transactions of the Royal Society of London Series B-Biological Sciences, 356*(1413), 1375–1384.

Conway M. A., & Holmes, E. A. (in press). Autobiographical memory and the working self. In N. R. Braisby & A. R. H. Gellatly (Eds.), *Cognitive psychology* (Ch. 14). Oxford: Oxford University Press.

Conway, M. A., Meares, K., & Standart, S. (2004). Images and goals. *Memory, 12*, 525–531.

Conway, M. A., & Pleydell-Pearce, C. W. (2000). The construction of autobiographical memories in the self-memory system. *Psychology Review, 107*(2), 261–288.

Dadds, M. R., Bovbjerg, D. H., Redd, W. H., & Cotmore, T. R. H. (1997). Imagery in classical conditioning. *Psychological Bulletin, 122*, 89–103.

Dadds, M. A., Hawes, D., Smith, B., & Vaka, C. (2004). Imagery and conditioning as a factor in psychopathology. *Memory 12*, 462–466.

Davey, G. C. (1989). UCS revaluation and conditioning models of acquired fears. *Behaviour Research and Therapy, 27*(5), 521–528.

Davey, G. C., de Jong, P. J. & Tallis, F. (1993). UCS inflation in the aetiology of a variety of anxiety disorders: Some case histories. *Behaviour Research and Therapy, 31*, 495–498.

Day, S., Holmes, E. A., & Hackmann, A. (2004). Occurrence of imagery and its links to memory in agoraphobia. *Memory, 12*, 416–427.

de Silva, P. (1986). Obsessional-compulsive imagery. *Behaviour Research and Therapy, 24*, 333–350.

Ehlers, A., & Clark, D. M. (2000). A cognitive model of posttraumatic stress disorder. *Behaviour Research and Therapy, 38*(4), 319–345.

Ehlers, A., Clark, D. M., Hackmann, A., McManus, F. & Fennell, M. J. V. (in press). Cognitive therapy for posttraumatic stress disorder: Development and evaluation. *Behaviour Research and Therapy.*

Ehlers, A., Clark, D. M., Hackmann, A., McManus, F., Fennell, M., Herbert, C. et al. (2003). A randomized controlled trial of cognitive therapy, self-help booklet, and repeated assessment as early interventions for PTSD. *Archives of General Psychiatry, 60*, 1024–1032.

Ehlers, A., Hackmann, A., & Michael, T. (2004). Intrusive re-experiencing in post-traumatic stress disorder: Phenomenology, theory, and therapy. *Memory, 12*, 403–415.

Ehlers, A., Hackmann, A., Steil, R., Clohessy, S., Wenninger, K., & Winter, H. (2002). The nature of intrusive memories after trauma: The warning signal hypothesis. *Behaviour Research and Therapy, 40*(9), 995–1002.

Foa, E. B., & Kozak, M. J. (1986). Emotional processing of fear: Exposure to corrective information. *Psychological Bulletin, 99*(1), 20–35.

Foa, E. B., Molnar, C., & Cashman, L. (1995). Change in rape narratives during exposure therapy for posttraumatic stress disorder. *Journal of Traumatic Stress, 8*(4), 675–690.

Foa, E. B., & Rothbaum, B. O. (1998). *Treating the trauma of rape: Cognitive-behavior therapy for PTSD.* New York: Guilford Press.

Gilbert, P., & Irons, C. (2004). A pilot exploration of the use of compassionate images in a group of self-critical people. *Memory, 12*, 507–516.

Grey, N., Holmes, E., & Brewin, C. (2001). It is not only fear: Peri-traumatic emotional hot spots in posttraumatic stress disorder. *Behavioural and Cognitive Psychotherapy, 29*(3), 367–372.

Grey, N., Young, K., & Holmes, E. (2002). Cognitive restructuring within reliving: A treatment for peritraumatic emotional "hotspots" in posttraumatic stress disorder. *Behavioural and Cognitive Psychotherapy, 30*(1), 37–56.

Hackmann, A. (1998). Working with images in clinical psychology. In A. S. Bellack & M. Hersen (Eds.), *Comprehensive Clinical Psychology, 6*(14), 301–318.

Hackmann, A., Clark, D. M., & McManus, F. (2000). Recurrent images and early memories in social phobia. *Behaviour Research and Therapy, 38*(6), 601–610.

Hackmann, A., Ehlers, A., Speckens, A., & Clark, D. M. (in press). Characteristics and content of intrusive memories in PTSD and their changes with treatment. *Journal of Traumatic Stress.*

Hackmann, A., Surawy, C., & Clark, D. M. (1998). Seeing yourself through others' eyes: A study of spontaneously occurring images in social phobia. *Behavioral and Cognitive Psychotherapy, 26,* 3–12.

HarperCollins (1995). *Collins English Dictionary* (3rd ed.). London: HarperCollins.

Harvey, A. G., Clark, D. M., Ehlers, A., & Rapee, R. (2000). Social anxiety and self impression: Cognitive preparation enhances the beneficial effects of video feedback following a stressful social task. *Behaviour Research and Therapy, 38*(12), 1183–1192.

Harvey, A., Watkins, E., Mansell, W., & Shafran, R. (in press). *Cognitive behavioural processes across psychological disorders: A transdiagnostic perspective to research and treatment.* Oxford: Oxford University Press.

Hirsch, C., Clark, D. M., Mathews, A., & Williams, R. (2003). Self-images play a causal role in social phobia. *Behaviour Research and Therapy, 41*(8), 909–921.

Hirsch, C., Meynen, T., & Clark, D. M. (2004). Negative self-imagery in social anxiety contaminates social interactions. *Memory, 12,* 496–506.

Holmes, E.A. (in press). Intrusive, emotional mental imagery and trauma: Experimental and clinical clues. *Imagination, Cognition and Personality.*

Holmes, E. A., Brewin, C. R., & Hennessy, R. G. (2004). Trauma films, information processing, and intrusive memory development. *Journal of Experimental Psychology: General, 133,* 3–22.

Holmes, E. A., Creswell, C., & O'Connor, T. G. (2004). *Post-traumatic stress symptoms in London school children following September 11th 2001: Peritraumatic reactions and imagery.* Manuscript submitted for publication.

Holmes, E. A., Grey, N., & Young, K. A. D. (in press). Intrusive images and "hotspots" of trauma memories in posttraumatic stress disorder: An exploratory investigation of emotions and cognitive themes. *Behavior Therapy and Experimental Psychiatry.*

Holmes, E. A., & Hackmann, A. (Eds.). (2004). Mental imagery and memory in psychopathology [special issue]. *Memory, 12,* 385–536.

Holmes, E. A., & Steel, C. (2004). Schizotypy: A vulnerability factor for traumatic intrusions. *Journal of Nervous and Mental Disease, 192,* 28–34.

Johnson, M. K. (1983). A multiple-entry, modular memory system. In G. H. Bower (Ed.), *The psychology of learning and motivation: Advances in research and theory* (Vol. 17, pp. 81–123). New York: Academic Press.

Kavanagh, D. J., Freese, S., Andrade, J., & May, J. (2001). Effects of visuospatial tasks on desensitization to emotive memories. *British Journal of Clinical Psychology, 40,* 267–280.

Kuyken, W., & Brewin, C. R. (1994). Autobiographical memory functioning in depression and reports of early abuse. *Journal of Abnormal Psychology, 104*(4), 585–591.

Lang, P. (1977). Imagery in therapy: An information processing analysis of fear. *Behaviour Therapy, 8,* 862–886.

Libby, L. K., & Eibach R. P. (2002). Looking back in time: Self-concept change affects visual perspective in autobiographical memory. *Journal of Personality and Social Psychology, 82,* 167–179.

Mansell, W. (2000). Conscious appraisal and the modification of automatic processes in anxiety. *Behavioural and Cognitive Psychotherapy, 28,* 99–120.

Mansell, W., & Lam, D. (2004). A preliminary study of autobiographical memory in remitted bipolar and unipolar depression. *Memory, 12,* 437–446.

Martin, M., & Williams, R. (1990). Imagery and emotion: Clinical and experimental approaches. In P. Hampson, P. J. Marks, F. David, & J. T. E. Richardson (Eds.), *Imagery: Current Developments* (pp. 268–306). Florence, KY: Taylor & Francis/Routledge.

May, J. (2003). *Images of desire.* Paper presented at the British Association for the Advancement of Science's Festival of Science, University of Salford, UK, September 11th.

May, J., Andrade, J., Panabokke, N., & Kavanagh, D. (2004). Images of desire: Cognitive models of craving. *Memory, 12,* 447–461.

McNally, R. J., Lasko, N. B., Macklin, M. L., & Pitman, R. K. (1995). Autobiographical memory disturbance in combat-related post-traumatic stress disorder. *Behaviour Research and Therapy, 33,* 619–630.

Morrison, A. P. (2001). The interpretation of intrusions in psychosis: An integrative cognitive approach to hallucinations and delusions. *Behavioural and Cognitive Psychotherapy, 29,* 257–276.

Morrison, A. P. (2004). The use of imagery in cognitive therapy for psychosis: A case example. *Memory, 12,* 517–524.

Morrison, A. P., & Baker, C. A. (2000). Intrusive thoughts and auditory hallucinations: A comparative study of intrusions in psychosis. *Behaviour Research and Therapy, 38*(11), 1097–1106.

Morrison, A. P., Beck, A. T., Glentworth, D., Dunn, H., Reid, G. S., & Larkin, W. (2002). Imagery and psychotic symptoms: A preliminary investigation. *Behaviour Research and Therapy, 40*(9), 1053–1062.

Mowrer, O. H. (1977) Mental imagery: An indispensible concept. *Journal of Mental Imagery, 1,* 303–325.

Nelson, J., & Harvey, A. (2002). The differential functions of imagery and verbal thought in insomnia. *Journal of Abnormal Psychology, 111,* 665–669.

Osman, S., Cooper, M., Veale, D., & Hackmann, A. (2004). An investigation into the nature and meaning of spontaneously occurring images in people with body dysmorphic disorder. *Memory, 12,* 428–436.

Panabokke, N., May, J., Eade, D., Andrade, J., & Kavanagh, D. (2004). *Visual imagery tasks suppress craving for cigarettes.* Manuscript submitted for publication.

Paivio, A. (1986). *Mental representation: A dual coding approach.* Oxford: Oxford University Press.

Pratt, D., Cooper, M., & Hackmann, A. (in press). Imagery and its characteristics in people who are anxious about spiders. *Behavioural and Cognitive Psychotherapy.*

Rachman, S. (1980). Emotional processing. *Behaviour Research and Therapy*, *18*, 51–60.

Roth, A., & Fonagy, P. (1996). *What works for whom? A critical review of psychotherapy research.* New York: Guilford Press.

Salkovskis, P. M. (2002). Empirically grounded clinical interventions: Cognitive behavioural therapy progresses through a multi-dimensional approach to clinical science. *Behavioural and Cognitive Psychotherapy*, *30*, 3–10.

Scott, J., Stanton, B., Garland, A., & Ferrier, I. N. (2000). Cognitive vulnerability in patients with bipolar disorder. *Psychological Medicine*, *30*, 467–472.

Speckens, A. (2003). *Imagery and early traumatic memories in obsessive-compulsive disorder.* Paper presented at the 31st annual conference of the British Association for Behavioural and Cognitive Psychotherapy. University of York, UK, July.

Steel, C., Fowler, D., & Holmes, E. A. (2004). *Trauma related intrusions in psychosis: An information processing account.* Manuscript submitted for publication.

Stopa, L., & Bryant, T. (2004). Memory perspective and self-concept: An exploratory study. *Memory*, *12*, 489–495.

Teasdale, J. D. (1999). Multi-level theories of cognition–emotion relations. In T. Dalgleish & M. J. Power (Eds.), *Handbook of cognition and emotion* (pp. 665–682). Chichester, UK: Wiley.

van der Kolk, B. A., & Fisler, R. (1995). Dissociation and the fragmentary nature of traumatic memories: Overview and exploratory study. *Journal of Traumatic Stress*, *8*(4), 505–525.

Wells, A., & Hackmann, A. (1993). Imagery and core beliefs in health anxiety: Content and origins. *Behavioural and Cognitive Therapy*, *21*, 265–273.

Williams, J. M. G., Healy, H. G., & Ellis, N. C. (1999). The effect of imageability and predictability of cues in autobiographical memory. *Quarterly Journal of Experimental Psychology*, *52*A, 555–579.

Williams, J. M. G., & Scott, J. (1998). Autobiographical memory in depression. *Psychological Medicine*, *18*, 689–695.

MEMORY, 2004, *12* (4), 403–415

Intrusive re-experiencing in post-traumatic stress disorder: Phenomenology, theory, and therapy

Anke Ehlers

Institute of Psychiatry, London, UK,

Ann Hackmann

University of Oxford, UK

Tanja Michael

University of Basle, Switzerland

The article describes features of trauma memories in post-traumatic stress disorder (PTSD), including characteristics of unintentional re-experiencing symptoms and intentional recall of trauma narratives. *Re-experiencing symptoms* are usually sensory impressions and emotional responses from the trauma that appear to lack a time perspective and a context. The vast majority of intrusive memories can be interpreted as re-experiencing of warning signals, i.e., stimuli that signalled the onset of the trauma or of moments when the meaning of the event changed for the worse. Triggers of re-experiencing symptoms include stimuli that have perceptual similarity to cues accompanying the traumatic event. *Intentional recall* of the trauma in PTSD may be characterised by confusion about temporal order, and difficulty in accessing important details, both of which contribute to problematic appraisals. Recall tends to be disjointed. When patients with PTSD deliberately recall the worst moments of the trauma, they often do not access other relevant (usually subsequent) information that would correct impressions/predictions made at the time. A theoretical analysis of re-experiencing symptoms and their triggers is offered, and implications for treatment are discussed. These include the need to actively incorporate updating information ("*I know now ...*") into the worst moments of the trauma memory, and to train patients to discriminate between the stimuli that were present during the trauma ("*then*") and the innocuous triggers of re-experiencing symptoms ("*now*").

Intrusive re-experiencing is a core symptom of post-traumatic stress disorder (PTSD). It can take various forms, including intrusive images, flashbacks, nightmares, and distress and physiological reactions when confronted with reminders (American Psychiatric Association, 1994). Surprisingly, relatively little is known about the phenomenology of re-experiencing (for reviews see

Reynolds & Brewin, 1998, 1999). Theorists concur in assuming that re-experiencing symptoms are due to the way trauma memories are encoded, organised in memory, and retrieved (e.g., Brewin, Dalgleish, & Joseph, 1996; Conway & Pleydell-Pearce, 2000; Ehlers & Clark, 2000; Foa & Rothbaum, 1998; Foa, Steketee, & Rothbaum, 1989; Keane, Zimmerling, & Caddell, 1985; van der

Correspondence should be sent to Professor Anke Ehlers, Department of Psychology (PO Box 77), Institute of Psychiatry, De Crespigny Park, Denmark Hill, London SE5 8AF, UK. Email: a.ehlers @ iop.kcl.ac.uk

The work described in this paper was funded by the Wellcome Trust. We thank Anne Speckens and the anonymous reviewers for their helpful comments.

© 2004 Psychology Press Ltd

http://www.tandf.co.uk/journals/pp/09658211.html   DOI:10.1080/09658210444000025

Kolk & Fisler, 1995). However, there is considerable debate as to what the core features of trauma memories are.

In this paper, we will describe characteristics of intrusive re-experiencing and of the intentional recall of trauma memories in post-traumatic stress disorder (PTSD) that our research group have identified from systematic interviews with trauma survivors with PTSD, from treating trauma survivors with cognitive behavioural therapy,[1] and from initial empirical studies. We hope to show that a detailed look at the phenomenology of trauma memories has implications for the theoretical explanation and treatment of PTSD.

QUALITIES OF INTRUSIVE RE-EXPERIENCING

Thoughts versus sensation

In the early literature on PTSD, it was not uncommon to describe intrusive memories as intrusive thoughts. This is a misleading term, as research suggests that intrusive (spontaneously triggered, unwanted) memories mainly consist of relatively brief sensory fragments of the traumatic experience (Ehlers & Steil, 1995; Mellman & Davis, 1985; van der Kolk & Fisler, 1995).

> Examples 1 and 2: A man kept seeing headlights coming towards him (as he had seen them shortly before his head-on car crash); a rape victim was haunted by images of the assailant's eyes starring through the letterbox (as she had seen them before the assailant broke into her house)

Ehlers and Steil (1995), Ehlers, Hackmann, Steil, Clohessy, Wenninger, and Winter (2002), and Hackmann, Ehlers, Speckens, and Clark (in press) found that, regardless of the type of trauma, visual sensations were most common, followed by other sensory impressions (bodily sensations, sounds, smells, and tastes). It was not uncommon for intrusive *memories* to have several sensory components, but they were rarely described as thoughts. The above data were collected in specifically probing for repetitive unwanted

memories about the trauma using instructions such as:

> After a traumatic event, many people have memories of the event that pop into their mind WHEN THEY DO NOT WANT THEM TO. Parts of the event may come to mind again and again. These are different for everyone. Do you have such unwanted memories that keep coming back?

Recent theoretical work suggests that intrusive memories should be distinguished from other non-memory cognitions that may also be experienced as intrusive, as these may be functionally distinct (Ehlers & Clark, 2000; Joseph, Williams, & Yule, 1997). Non-memory intrusive cognitions include evaluative thoughts about the trauma that may actually be more frequent than intrusive images or flashbacks (Reynolds & Brewin, 1998, 1999), and rumination (e.g., "Why did it happen to me?", "How could the event have been prevented?", or dwelling on how one's life has been ruined by the trauma) which is common in PTSD and is an important maintaining factor (Murray, Ehlers & Mayou, 2002). Past research has not always separated intrusive memories from rumination (e.g., Holman & Silver, 1998).

Lack of time perspective

Memories of specific autobiographical events are usually discussed in the literature as episodic memories, a concept introduced by Tulving to describe a memory system that makes possible the acquisition and retrieval of information about specific experiences that occurred at a particular time and place (see Tulving, 2002). Retrieval from episodic memory is unique in that it involves autonoetic awareness (the sense or experience of the self in the past).

The intrusive re-experiencing symptoms in PTSD appear to lack one of the defining features of episodic memories, the awareness that the content of the memory is *something from the past*. In a dissociative flashback the individual loses all awareness of present surroundings, and literally appears to relive the experience. The sensory impressions are re-experienced as if they were features of something happening right now, rather than being aspects of memories from the past. Also, the emotions (including physical reactions and motor responses) accompanying them are the same as those experienced at the time ("original"

---

[1] We will give case examples illustrating our observations from these studies. These summarise the descriptions given by the patient, and in some cases include links that the therapist made (e.g., between triggers and intrusive memories). Details of some of the examples are modified to prevent identification of patients, however, all important facts are accurate.

emotions) (Brewin et al., 1996; Ehlers & Clark, 2000; Foa & Rothbaum, 1998).

> Example 3: A woman who had been attacked by a bull saw a number plate with the letters "MOO" at a petrol station. This triggered a flashback during which she re-experienced the impending attack, and sprayed another customer with diesel fuel. At this time she was totally unaware that what she was experiencing involved material from memory.

In a less dramatic form, the lack of time perspective also appears to apply to other forms of re-experiencing, including intrusive images or distress in response to reminders. Patients may not lose all awareness of present surroundings, but their intrusions are accompanied by a sense of current threat and a sense of "nowness", i.e., the feeling that the sensations are experienced in the present rather than a memory from the past. Re-experiencing includes a phenomenon that Ehlers and Clark (2000) termed *affect without recollection*. Individuals with PTSD sometimes re-experience physiological sensations or emotions that were associated with the traumatic event *without* a recollection of the event itself (lack of source information, see Schacter, Norman, & Koutstaal, 1997; see also classical conditioning interpretations below).

> Example 4: A rape victim noticed that she was feeling extremely anxious while talking to a female friend in a restaurant, and only subsequently realised that the feeling was probably triggered by the presence of a man nearby who bore some physical resemblance to the rapist.

Lack of context

Van der Kolk and van der Hart (1991) suggested that intrusive trauma memories are relatively invulnerable to change. In line with this suggestion, Hackmann et al. (in press) systematically interviewed patients with PTSD about their intrusive memories and found that each patient experienced a small number of intrusions that occurred in a stereotyped, repetitive way. Ehlers and Clark (2000) observed that PTSD sufferers re-experience their original emotions and sensory impressions even if they later (either during the event or afterwards) acquire new information that contradicts the original impression.

> Example 5: A patient whose father committed suicide by shooting himself, kept re-experiencing a panicky urge to find him, and the feeling of responsibility for rescuing him that he had when he discovered the suicide note. At the time, he erroneously thought his father had taken sleeping tablets and could be saved if he acted quickly.

Of particular interest for understanding intrusive re-experiencing is the observation that patients may even have two intrusions that contradict each other, without any change in these intrusions over time.

> Example 6: A woman whose daughter died in a house fire while she was out, had frequent horrifying intrusions of seeing the curtains burning when she returned. She had assumed when she saw the curtains that her daughter was burning alive. However, she subsequently discovered that the daughter had been upstairs, and had been overcome by fumes. For many years, the patient experienced daily intrusions of the curtains burning. She also had intrusions of seeing the body of her daughter in the mortuary, with no sign of burns. Before treatment, she had never connected these two parts of the memory for the traumatic event.

As the example shows, when an intrusive memory is triggered, people with PTSD do not seem able to put it into context, and appear unable to access information that corrected or updated the impression and feelings they had at the time (e.g., the fact that the daughter did not burn alive), probably contributing to the lack of time perspective described above (see also Koriat, Goldsmith & Pansky, 2000).

Which of the intrusion characteristics predict PTSD?

In the initial aftermath of trauma, intrusive re-experiencing is common. Shalev (1992) found that the presence of these symptoms is not a good predictor of PTSD. Are certain characteristics of intrusive memories better at predicting PTSD than the presence of initial re-experiencing symptoms? Michael (2000) conducted two studies of assault survivors. Several characteristics of intrusive memories distinguished between survivors with and without PTSD and predicted subsequent PTSD severity. These included: distress caused by the intrusion; lack of time perspective (operationalised by the degree to which the intrusion was experienced as something happening "now"); and lack of context (operationalised by the degree to which it was experienced as isolated and disconnected from what happened before and afterwards) (for further predictors such as the interpretation of the intrusive memories see Ehlers & Steil, 1995; Steil & Ehlers, 2000).

CONTENT OF INTRUSIVE MEMORIES

Ehlers et al. (2002) examined the content of intrusive memories and found that they do not appear to be random fragments. They mainly represented stimuli that signalled the *onset* of the trauma or of the moments with the largest emotional impact. Ehlers et al. (2002) argued that they can be understood as stimuli that—through *temporal* association with the traumatic event—acquired the status of warning signals: stimuli that, if encountered again, would indicate impending danger. This would explain why intrusive memories induce a sense of serious current threat, as Ehlers and Clark (2000) suggested.

> Example 7: A woman who was raped in her home kept seeing the perpetrator standing inside her bedroom door as she had seen him when she woke up (before she was attacked).

The warning signal interpretation of intrusive memories was inspired by initial observations that intrusive memories did not appear to represent a simple replaying of the most distressing moments. For example, on the basis of research showing that central elements of highly emotional experiences are remembered best (Christianson, 1992a), one may have expected the rape survivor in Example 7 to re-experience sensations from the most distressing moments of her ordeal, for example, the taste connected with having to perform oral sex on the perpetrator—rather than the sight of the perpetrator *before* she was attacked.

The warning signal hypothesis extends previous attempts to explain re-experiencing with conditioning theories (e.g., Charney, Deutch, Krystal, Southwick, & Davis, 1993; Keane et al., 1985; Kilpatrick & Veronen, 1983; for a review of the role of imagery in human classical conditioning see Dadds, Bovbjerg, & Redd, 1997) in that it is designed to explain the particular content of intrusive memories. Classical conditioning theory

may facilitate prediction of the kinds of warning signals that will be re-experienced (e.g., processes of temporal contiguity and predictive significance).

It is important to note that the "warning" stimuli reflect temporal association, rather than necessarily having a meaningful relationship to the trauma. Many seem to consist of markers of the situational context in which the trauma occurred. Markers of location may be understood as early warning signals that can be spotted from far away and avoided in the future.

> Example 8: A man who witnessed the suicide of a person who jumped in front of a train re-experienced the sight of railway tracks as he had seen them before the person jumped. He did not re-experience the sight of the train approaching, which had a closer relationship in meaning to the suicide.

In prolonged trauma, there may be several crucial moments when meanings change for the worse, each of which can be represented in re-experiencing. Furthermore, moments with the largest emotional impact do not necessarily occur during the trauma itself, but may occur later when the patient realises what could have happened, or when something gives the situation a more traumatic personal meaning. Ehlers et al. (2002) observed that even for intrusions that relate to moments during the course of the traumatic event or its aftermath, the content of the intrusion seems to follow the warning signal hypothesis. Like intrusions of stimuli that preceded the onset of the trauma, these intrusions appear to be mainly of stimuli that signalled a change in meaning to the worse, including stimuli that are not necessarily meaningfully related to this change.

> Example 9: A woman re-experienced a touch on her shoulder. After her accident she had been trapped in her car, but initially did not realise that she was hurt. A paramedic had touched her shoulder and asked whether she was all right. It was following this question that she felt pain and realised that she could be badly hurt.

Hackmann et al. (in press) subjected the warning signal hypothesis to an empirical test. They systematically interviewed PTSD patients about their intrusive memories and classified their content. Patients were asked to identify their main intrusion. A total of 92% of the patients' main intrusions could be classified as warning signals.

These either signalled the onset of the trauma (e.g., "perpetrator standing with a knife next to my bed" in a patient subsequently assaulted with the knife, 55%), or signalled a moment when the meaning of the event became more traumatic (e.g., "seeing two policemen standing next to my bed"—the policemen later told the patient that others had died in the accident, 37%).

TRIGGERS OF RE-EXPERIENCING SYMPTOMS

Many theorists of PTSD have commented on the wide range of triggers of involuntary re-experiencing (e.g., Brewin et al., 1996; Ehlers & Clark, 2000; Foa et al., 1989). Most individuals with PTSD report that newspaper or TV reports of similar events provoke intrusions. Many report wide-ranging generalisation of fear to stimuli only loosely connected to the original traumatic stimulus (see Example 3).

Furthermore, as Ehlers and Clark (2000) observed, many of the trigger stimuli are cues that do *not* have a *strong meaningful* relationship to the traumatic event, but instead are simply cues that were *temporally associated* with the event (see also Charney et al., 1993; Keane et al., 1985), for example physical cues similar to those present shortly before or during the trauma (e.g., a pattern of light, a tone of voice); or matching internal cues (e.g., touch on a certain part of the body, proprioceptive feedback from one's own movements). People with PTSD are usually unaware of these triggers, so intrusions appear to come out of the blue. Ehlers et al. (2002) observed that triggers of intrusive memories are often stimuli that bear physical resemblance to stimuli that immediately preceded the "warning signal" that is later re-experienced (Example 11), or to the "warning signal" itself (Example 10).

Example 10: A car crash survivor was relaxing in his garden when he suddenly became very anxious and had intrusions of headlights coming towards him. Only later he realised that these were triggered by a bright patch of sunlight on his lawn.

Example 11: A woman whose car had been hit from behind, experienced intrusions of blue and yellow colours accompanied by strong fear when she was washing up and turned to the left to get the tea towel. After the impact, she had turned left to see what was happening and had seen that a

blue and yellow bus had hit her car. Turning to the right did not trigger intrusions.

FEATURES OF INTENTIONAL RECALL OF TRAUMA MEMORIES

The memory fragmentation debate

Several theorists have suggested that trauma memories are different from other auto-biographical memories (e.g., Brewin et al., 1996; Ehlers & Clark, 2000; Foa et al., 1989). For example, van der Kolk and Fisler (1995, p. 513) postulated that trauma memories are initially recollected in a sensory form "without any semantic representation ... experienced primarily as fragments of the sensory components of the event". Accordingly, several theorists have argued that one of the functions of PTSD treatment is the creation of an organised narrative with a beginning, middle, and end (e.g., Foa & Rothbaum, 1998; van der Kolk & Fisler, 1995).

Some studies have attempted to assess the degree of fragmentation by coding deliberately retrieved narrative accounts of traumatic events. Indices of fragmentation correlated with the severity of PTSD symptoms in cross-sectional (Amir, Stafford, Freshman, & Foa, 1998; Harvey & Bryant, 1999; Koss, Figueredo, Bell, Tharan, & Tromp, 1996), and prospective longitudinal studies (Halligan, Michael, Clark, & Ehlers, 2003). Foa, Molnar, and Cashman (1995) reported that patients' narrative accounts become more organised with exposure treatment, although not all changes in fragmentation indices are necessarily specific to patients who show clinical improvement (van der Minnen, 2002). Furthermore, Tromp, Koss, Figueredo, and Tharan (1995) recruited rape survivors and found that in contrast to other unpleasant and pleasant memories, accounts of rape memories were less clear, less vivid, and less detailed.

Critics of the memory fragmentation concept have argued that the so-called fragmentation of trauma memories is not surprising because in every autobiographical memory encoding is incomplete, and memory is always a reconstruction rather than an exact record (e.g., McNally, 2003). McNally (2003) points out that much about trauma memories can be explained by Easterbrook's (1959) finding that the focus of attention narrows during stress, and people appear to zoom in on central aspects, at the expense of remembering peripheral details (Christianson, 1992a). As trauma is a period of extreme stress, one might expect people only to encode the most important elements, rather than blow-by-blow minutiae. And one would expect that the most important elements are remembered very well, as high levels of stress usually enhance rather than impair memory (Shobe & Kihlstrom, 1997).

Consistent with these critical evaluations of the fragmentation concept, nearly all trauma survivors seen by our research team remember the gist of what happened well (e.g., that they have been stabbed, or had a car crash), but show confusion about or inability to access some details, and are often unclear about the exact temporal order of the events. This in itself is not surprising, as many memories of other events have similar characteristics. For example, people remember the gist of what was said at a meeting rather than a word-by-word record of who said what. However, people do not usually have persistent intrusive memories of meetings. The crucial question remains why people with PTSD have persistent re-experiencing symptoms, and what aspects of trauma memories explain them.

The debate about memory fragmentation has been complicated by the inconsistent use of the term in the literature. Van der Kolk and Fisler's description (1995) seems to characterise intrusive (i.e., unwanted, *automatically triggered*) trauma memories, and the phenomenology of re-experiencing symptoms as described above largely appears to be consistent with their description. Most research studies on memory fragmentation have investigated *intentional* recall in the form of trauma narratives.

Equating these two aspects of trauma memories would assume that they both reflect a single memory trace. We think that this is a problematic assumption. What is retrieved from memory about a traumatic event depends on the retrieval route and on the different memory processes/systems involved (see also Tulving, 2001). Thus, when describing characteristics of trauma memories, one has to bear in mind that they may only apply to certain retrieval routes and memory processes/systems.

A further problem with the research on memory fragmentation concerns assessment. In the empirical studies cited above, memory fragmentation was usually operationalised by coding trauma narratives for the proportion of utterances of confusion about what was happening, lack of organised thoughts, incomprehensible/muddled descriptions, or repetitions; by using global measures of readability or comprehensibility, or by self-report. Overall, the preliminary results in support of a fragmentation of trauma memories point to a deficit in the cohesion of narratives that is related to the severity of PTSD. Whether or not trauma narratives are also less detailed than narratives of other emotional events is less clear. Porter and Birt (2001) asked undergraduates to write down a description of their most traumatic memory as well as a description of a positive event, and rated the number of details in the narrative among other characteristics such as vividness of the memories. The traumatic memories actually contained more details than the positive memories, rather than fewer as one may have expected on the basis of the fragmentation idea. There was no difference in coherence ratings. The non-clinical sample and the possible ceiling effects in coherence ratings may compromise conclusions on trauma narratives. Nevertheless, trauma memories may not differ from other emotional memories in the overall number of details that can be accessed.

These studies illustrate that different indices of fragmentation may give different results. None of the measures used so far is satisfactory, as they either included irrelevant aspects (e.g., the overall number of details is less relevant than ability to recall detail that is important for the meaning of the event, see below) and/or did not assess relevant aspects (e.g., subtle gaps in memory). Readability of narratives may reflect characteristics of the survivor such as verbal intelligence or education rather than characteristics of the particular trauma memory (especially if trauma narratives are not compared to narratives of other emotional events; Gray & Lombardo, 2001). Utterances of confusion may represent problems at encoding rather than problems with retrieval from memory. In addition, the fragmentation indices are probably not sensitive enough in measuring the extent to which people with PTSD experience and remember their traumatic event as a *series* of *disjointed* events rather than *one* single event organised by a *time-line* (see Example 6). We think that this disjointedness of trauma memories is crucial in understanding re-experiencing (see below). Self-report measures such as the one used by Halligan et al. (2003) may assess different aspects of fragmentation more comprehensively, but are limited by their reliance on introspection.

A further important problem is that the fragmentation of the whole trauma narrative is less relevant for explaining re-experiencing than the fragmented recall of those time points that are later re-experienced.

Example 12: A patient appeared to have very coherent memory of a fatal car crash and reported that he could remember the accident in great detail, in a "frame by frame" fashion. His main intrusion was the sound of the crash. When he relived the event in therapy, he retrieved a detail that he had not remembered when thinking about the event before: After the impact (i.e., after the sound), he had seen the other driver collapsed over her steering wheel, realised she was dead, and thought he had killed her (although the accident was not his fault).

Similarly, Hellawell and Brewin (2002) distinguished between parts of trauma narratives that were like ordinary autobiographical memories, and parts that are accompanied by a marked sense of reliving, which they termed "flashback memories", and other authors have described as "hot spots" (i.e., most emotional points) during reliving (e.g., Ehlers & Clark, 2000; Foa & Rothbaum, 1998). A first empirical investigation that assessed hot spots and unintentional intrusive memories independently, did indeed find a close relationship (Holmes, Grey, & Young, 2003).

Thus, the most emotional parts of the intentional recall of the trauma are most relevant for the fragmentation debate, and for re-experiencing. We suggest that problems with what people with PTSD intentionally recall of the trauma may maintain PTSD in two ways: first, by affecting their appraisals of the event, and second, by preventing information stored in memory from being updated with subsequent information that corrects predictions (including a "felt sense" of what was going to happen) made at the time.

Influence of trauma recall on appraisals

Problematic appraisals of the traumatic event may be linked to different aspects of what people recall of the trauma (1) confusion about the time course of events, (2) problems in accessing important details of the event, (2) problematic recall stemming from encoding errors at the time of the event.

Confusion about the temporal order of an event can crucially affect its meaning and its implications for the future.

Example 13: A man who had been assaulted by a group of people developed a strong fear of being attacked again by people of the same ethnic group. His fear was dramatically reduced when he reconstructed the order of events and remembered that he had actually punched one of the group members first.

An inability to retrieve details of a traumatic event is not a problem if the detail is irrelevant for the meaning of the event. This will apply to many details of traumatic events as it does to details of memories of other events (McNally, 2003). However, our observations in treating patients with PTSD show that difficulty in accessing a particular detail can make a crucial difference for the personal meaning of the event.

Example 14: A patient who had been run over by a motorbike felt responsible, as she thought that if she had walked faster the bike would not have hit her. When visiting the site of the accident she remembered that the motorbike had actually tried to pass in front of her rather than behind her as she had assumed.

Furthermore, some patients do not even remember aspects that one would consider a central element of the experience.

Example 15: A rape victim was ashamed about complying with the perpetrator's instructions. When she relived the event in treatment she remembered that the assailant had threatened her with a knife. An objective observer would call the knife a central element, and as such it should be remembered well (Christianson, 1992a; Easterbrook, 1959), yet the patient did not initially access this information.

There are different interpretations of this phenomenon. First, one may argue that the inability to remember the knife was related to avoidance of thinking about the most frightening parts of the event. Second, the problem with the intentional recall of this central information may be related to problems at encoding, in that extreme arousal and/or confusion during trauma may compromise the differentiation of what is central and what is peripheral.

Similarly, during the traumatic event, individuals may not have enough cognitive capacity to decide that some very threatening aspects are not true, and thus encode them as real, or to encode the source of information accurately (see also Koriat et al., 2000).

Example 16: A rape victim remained convinced that she was unattractive because the rapist had repeatedly told her so. The extreme distress she experienced made it impossible for her to appreciate that this was simply a strategy that the rapist used to humiliate her.

Example 17: Some political prisoners start to believe that they are criminals after traumatic interrogations involving torture (Ehlers, Maercker & Boos, 2000).

This appears to include frightening images that people may experience during trauma. People with PTSD may respond to such images (and develop re-experiencing symptoms) as if they were a true part of the event, even if they later realised that they were an image rather than reality.

Example 18: A football fan was caught in a fight between football hooligans and the police. He had an image of the police smashing up his car and was terrified by this image. Subsequently, he developed flashbacks to the image and extreme anxiety when seeing police officers.

Disjointedness and lack of updating/linking to other information

When patients with PTSD initially relive the trauma in treatment, they appear to retrieve it in separate, disjointed parts, rather than as segments of an integrated memory. We have observed that when PTSD sufferers remember a particularly distressing segment ("hotspots"), they do not access other relevant (usually subsequent) information that corrected impressions they had or predictions they made at the time. (Note that the term prediction is used to include a "felt sense" of what might happen, not just conscious thoughts.)

Example 19: A patient who thought that he was going to die during an assault, and would never see his children again, was not able (whilst recalling this particularly distressing moment) to access the fact that he actually survived and still lived with his children. This part of the memory elicited overwhelming sadness.

The disjointedness in intentional recall of the most distressing parts of the traumatic experience ("hotspots") resembles the lack of context information that we described above as one of the characteristics of intrusive trauma memories. Our clinical observations suggest that the hotspots and intrusive memories are closely linked. A systematic study by Holmes et al. (in press) supports this view. Similarly, Holman and Silver (1998) observed that temporal disintegration at the time of the trauma—whereby the present moment becomes isolated from the continuity of past and present time—was associated with subsequent distress.

THEORETICAL EXPLANATION

Ehlers and Clark (2000) built on recent research on non-trauma autobiographical memories to explain re-experiencing symptoms. Despite an abundance of retrieval cues, people are usually not flooded by involuntary memories in their everyday life. As Conway and colleagues have demonstrated (e.g., Conway & Pleydell-Pearce, 2000), this is because autobiographical events are elaborated and incorporated into an autobiographical memory knowledge base. The elaboration enhances the ease of intentional retrieval through higher-order meaning-based retrieval strategies, and *inhibits* cued retrieval through direct triggering by stimuli associated with the event (see Conway & Pleydell-Pearce, 2000; Markowitsch, 1995). When an autobiographical memory enters consciousness, it comprises both specific information about the event *and* context information.

Ehlers and Clark (2000) proposed that in PTSD one of the problems is that trauma memories are not fully elaborated in this way (see also Brewin et al., 1996; Foa et al., 1989; Rachman, 1980). They are inadequately integrated into their context in time, place, and subsequent and previous information. This explains the problems described above with intentional recall, the "here and now" quality (no context in time), and the absence of links to subsequent information (e.g., "I did not die") described earlier. It also contributes to triggering by matching cues, as the inhibitory effect of elaboration is lacking.

In order to fully explain the easy triggering of re-experiencing symptoms, the wide range of triggers and the phenomenon of *affect without recollection*, Ehlers and Clark (2000) suggested that two further memory processes are involved: perceptual priming (enhanced ability to identify objects as a result of a prior encounter) and associative learning (see also Charney et al., 1993; Keane et al., 1985, Kilpatrick & Veronen, 1983). These two memory processes underlie *expectations* (note that we use this term more broadly than those involving conscious thoughts) about what stimuli the individual will encounter (priming) and what will happen next (associative learning). Together, they make it likely that the individual will notice external (e.g., visual or auditory cues) or internal (e.g., posture, feelings, arousal) stimulus configurations that are trauma reminders, and respond to them with automatically triggered re-experiencing symptoms.[2] Figure 1 illustrates how the combination of these processes leads to re-experiencing symptoms.

Ehlers and Clark (2000) proposed that people with PTSD have strong perceptual priming for stimuli that they encountered shortly before and during the trauma. There is a processing advantage and reduced perceptual threshold for these stimuli. Cues associated with the trauma that directly trigger memories of the event (as the inhibitory effect of elaboration/integration into context is lacking) are more likely to be noticed. Implicit memory traces are not well discriminated from other memory traces (Baddeley, 1997). Therefore vague physical similarity would be sufficient for the perception of stimuli as similar to those present during the trauma (poor stimulus discrimination) and thus for the triggering of intrusions, even if the context in which the stimulus configuration is observed is very different (see Example 10).[3]

In other cases, re-experiencing symptoms are connected to the trigger stimulus by associative learning (see Example 11). As retrieval from associative memory is cue-driven and unintentional, individuals may just experience the emotional response associated with the trigger stimulus, and may not always be aware that their emotional reaction is due to activation of the trauma memory (*affect without recollection*).

As discussed above, intrusive memories are usually of stimuli that can be understood as warning signals, stimuli that predicted the onset of the trauma, or a moment when meaning changed for the worse. These considerations show that re-experiencing symptoms "make sense" in that they can be understood as the result of processes that help to warn the organism of impending danger. Perceptual priming sets up the expectation that the individual may encounter again a stimulus configuration such as the one encountered shortly before/at the onset of the traumatic event or its worst moments. Associative learning serves to inform the individual what is likely to happen next, and trigger the corresponding emotional responses so that a behavioural response can be quickly activated.

The pattern of preferential identification of cues that resemble those predicting the traumatic event and strong emotional response to these triggers appears to be an adaptive response shortly after trauma, as the individual needs to re-evaluate the safety of his/her environment. Many people will quickly recover as they process the trauma, and establish an elaborated autobiographical memory for it. They notice that the triggers are false alarms and do not signal current threat. However, in some individuals re-experiencing will persist, for two reasons.[4]

First, if individuals fail to put the trauma memories into their context and update them with subsequent information (e.g., in Example 10, "I did not die in the head-on car crash, and I have seen headlights many of times before and after the crash without having an accident"), re-experiencing to trigger cues (bright spots in dark background) will persist (they will remain predictors of "I am going to die").

Second, individuals may not be aware of the triggers of re-experiencing symptoms. Failure to identify triggers makes it difficult for the patient to discriminate such triggers from the stimuli that

---

[2] See also Tulving's notion, 2001, 2002, that perceptual information from personal experience can be retrieved independent of the episodic memory system, without autonoetic remembering, and case examples of patients who do not have a memory of the trauma, but still show fear responses to reminders or intrusive images (e.g., Christianson, 1992b).

[3] Experimental studies from our laboratory have found that assault survivors with PTSD show stronger priming for traumatic material than those without PTSD (Michael, Ehlers, & Halligan, 2004). Furthermore, analogue studies have shown that stimuli occurring in a traumatic context were more strongly primed than stimuli occurring in a neutral context. Enhanced priming predicted the occurrence of PTSD-like intrusions (Michael & Ehlers, 2004). Thus, there is experimental evidence pointing to perceptual priming as one mechanism underlying intrusive memories in PTSD.

[4] Note that, in addition, the Ehlers and Clark (2000) model specifies other maintaining factors in PTSD, overly negative apprraisals of the trauma and/or it sequelae, and dysfunctional behaviours and cognitive strategies.

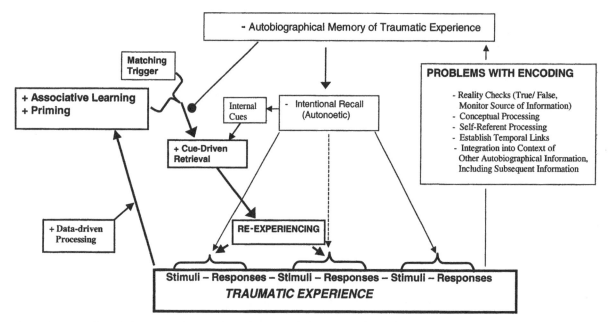

Figure 1. Encoding of the traumatic experience (arrows pointing upwards) and its retrieval from memory (arrows pointing downwards) in people with PTSD, according to the Ehlers and Clark (2000) model. Strong processes are indicated with +, bold printing, and fat arrows; weak or deficient processes with –, plain text, and thin arrows. Pointed arrows indicate facilitation, round arrows inhibition. Dashed arrows represent difficult access.

For simplification, the traumatic experience is presented as a series of stimuli and responses (including sensations, emotions, thoughts). People with PTSD show strong perceptual priming for stimuli that they perceived shortly before and during the trauma; and strong associative learning of stimulus–response or stimulus–stimulus patterns. On the other hand, problems with encoding the traumatic experience result in a poorly elaborated autobiographical memory for the event that is inadequately linked to other autobiographical information.

The three memory processes interact and lead to the easy triggering of re-experiencing symptoms: Strong perceptual priming (1) and associative learning (2) facilitate cue-driven retrieval to matching triggers. As the autobiographical memory is poorly elaborated (3), there is little inhibition of cue-driven retrieval of elements of the experience that lacks the context information of other autobiographical memories. Furthermore, intentional recall of parts of the experience may indirectly trigger re-experiencing symptoms by providing cues for cue-driven retrieval.

Intentional recall with autonoetic awareness may be hampered in several ways, depending on the nature of the encoding problems. Recall tends to be disjointed and relevant (usually subsequent) information may not be accessed when recalling the worst parts of the experience; recall may omit parts of the experience; there may be confusion about the order of events in time, or the source and truth-value of information; and the resulting recall may lack the perspective of time (see Examples 12 to 19 in text).

they encountered during the trauma, and to learn that there is no present danger.

IMPLICATIONS FOR TREATMENT

The study of intrusive and intentionally retrieved trauma memories, and their theoretical analysis, has led us to develop an effective version of cognitive behavioural therapy for PTSD (Ehlers & Clark, 2000). The treatment has been evaluated in two randomised controlled trials and shown to be highly effective (effect sizes of 2.5 and above in intent-to-treat analyses) and acceptable (overall drop-out rate across studies of less than 2%) (Ehlers et al., 2003, in press). The treatment disseminated well into a clinical trauma service, with similarly high effect sizes (Gillespie, Duffy,

Hackmann, & Clark, 2002). We will briefly describe the therapeutic strategies used to decrease re-experiencing symptoms. The interventions are based on the theoretical analysis described above. Other elements of the treatment not described here deal with problematic appraisals of the trauma and its sequelae, and with dysfunctional behaviours and cognitive strategies that maintain PTSD (see Ehlers & Clark, 2000).

Updating and integrating trauma memories

The features of recall of trauma memories in PTSD described above (difficulty in accessing important details, confusion about the order of events, difficulty in accessing information that updated impressions/predictions made at the time of the trauma, and disjointed recall), suggest that it is necessary for patients to reconstruct exactly what happened, after the trauma. For many trauma survivors, this happens during natural recovery, when they think over or discuss the experience. For those who do not recover spontaneously, the reconstruction and elaboration of what exactly happened during the traumatic event is an important treatment goal. Various effective ways of achieving this have been developed, e.g., repeated imaginal reliving (Foa & Rothbaum, 1998) or writing a trauma narrative (Resick & Schnicke, 1993).

Building on these techniques, Ehlers and Clark (2000) suggested that a particularly efficient way of updating trauma memories and putting them into their context is to (1) identify the moments during the trauma that create the greatest distress and sense of "nowness" during recall ("hotspots") through imaginal reliving (or writing a narrative) and discussion of intrusive memories, (2) identify information that updates the impression the patient had at the time either by identifying the course, circumstances, and outcome of the trauma or by cognitive restructuring, and (3) actively incorporate the updating information into the hot spots using verbal and imagery techniques.

Example 20: A motorbike rider was hit by a car. His main intrusion was of flying through the air. The intrusion was linked to the worst moment, which happened shortly afterwards, when he saw an image of himself in pieces and thought he was dead. In therapy, updating information was incorporated into the trauma narrative at the point when he had this image. This was first done by verbally reminding himself of the updating information "I now know I am alive and my body is complete" and by touching his legs and body when coming to this point. Furthermore, the patient did an image transformation of joining his body together and getting up from the ground.

Grey, Young, and Holmes (2002) have recently elaborated on therapeutic techniques to achieve the incorporation of updating information.

Identifying and discriminating triggers of intrusions

As described above, patients with PTSD are often not aware of perceptual cues that trigger intrusive memories. Education and training in the identification of triggers and stimulus discrimination is helpful. Patients need to learn the discrimination between the "then" and the "now", i.e., the present stimuli that trigger intrusions and those encountered during the trauma. They need to learn to realise when they encounter these stimuli that these are just reminders of the event and do not indicate danger now, as they occur in a different context. In our treatment protocol (Ehlers & Clark, 2000), patients are instructed to observe triggers of intrusive memories, and to pay close attention to the differences between the harmless trigger and its present context ("now") and the stimulus configuration that occurred in the context of trauma ("then"). It can be useful to instruct the patient to repeatedly bring on intrusive memories to practise this discrimination.

Example 21: A woman who had been raped experienced flashbacks when attempting intercourse with her partner. In therapy, the similarities and differences between the ways the rapist ("then") and her partner ("now") touched her and the context of these sensations were highlighted, and she practised staying aware of the differences when being with her partner.

CONCLUSIONS

This paper has shown that it is important to consider features of unintentional and intentional recall when characterising trauma memories in PTSD. Laboratory experiments on eyewitness testimony using paradigms requiring intentional recall had suggested that central elements of traumatic experiences should be remembered best (Christianson, 1992a; McNally, 2003), and that details may be remembered less well. While this pattern is overall consistent with the trauma narratives given by patients with PTSD, it does not explain the content of re-experiencing symptoms. A warning signal interpretation appears to fit their content better. Furthermore, problems with what is intentionally recalled contribute to problematic appraisals of the trauma, and are thus important in understanding the psychopathology of PTSD. Investigations into the phenomenology of intrusive memories and intentional recall of trauma memories led to a new theoretical model and treatment approach. A central element of treatment involves the active incorporation of information that updates and corrects the predictions made at the worst moments of the trauma through verbal and imagery techniques. This information is either derived from knowledge of how the event and its consequences unfolded, or on cognitive restructuring of misperceptions and misinterpretations. Other CBT approaches have either relied on repeated exposure to the trauma narrative or on cognitive restructuring outside the imaginal exposure to deal with the worst moments of the trauma. In our experience, the active integration of the updating/corrective information into the trauma memory is usually necessary for the patient to achieve full benefit from the intervention. This observation matches the finding that before treatment patients do not access the updating/corrective information when remembering the worst moments, as the trauma appears to be retrieved as disjointed segments that are inadequately integrated into their context.

REFERENCES

American Psychiatric Association (1994). *Diagnostic and statistical manual of mental disorders* (4th ed.). Washington, DC: Author.

Amir, N., Stafford, J., Freshman, M. S., & Foa, E. B. (1998). Relationship between trauma narratives and trauma pathology. *Journal of Traumatic Stress, 11*, 385–392.

Baddeley, A. (1997). *Human memory. Theory and practice* (Rev. ed.). Hove, UK: Psychology Press.

Brewin, C. R., Dalgleish, T., & Joseph, S. (1996). A dual representation theory of posttraumatic stress disorder. *Psychological Review, 103*, 670–686.

Charney, D. S., Deutch, A. Y., Krystal, J. H., Southwick, S. M., & Davis, M. (1993). Psychobiologic mechanisms of posttraumatic stress disorder. *Archives of General Psychiatry, 50*, 294–305.

Christianson, S. A. (1992a). Emotional stress and eyewitness memory: A critical review. *Psychological Bulletin, 112*, 284–309.

Christianson, S. A. (1992b). Remembering emotional events: Potential mechanisms. In S. A. Christianson (Ed.), *The handbook of emotion and memory: Research and theory*. Hillsdale, NJ: Lawrence Erlbaum Associates Inc.

Conway, M. A., & Pleydell-Pearce, C. W. (2000). The construction of autobiographical memories in the self-memory system. *Psychological Review, 27*, 261–286.

Dadds, M. R., Bovbjerg, D. H., & Redd, W. H. (1997) Imagery in human classical conditioning. *Psychological Bulletin, 122*, 89–103.

Easterbrook, J. A. (1959). The effect of emotion on cue utilization and the organisation of behavior. *Psychological Review, 66*, 183–201.

Ehlers, A., & Clark, D. M. (2000). A cognitive model of posttraumatic stress disorder. *Behaviour Research and Therapy, 38*, 319–345.

Ehlers, A., Clark, D. M., Hackmann, A., McManus F., & Fennell, M. (in press). Cognitive therapy for PTSD: Development and evaluation. *Behavior Research and Therapy*.

Ehlers, A., Clark, D. M., Hackmann, A., McManus F., Fennell, M., Herbert, C., & Mayou, R. (2003). A randomized controlled trial of cognitive therapy, self-help booklet, and repeated assessment as early interventions for PTSD. *Archives of General Psychiatry, 60*, 1024–1032.

Ehlers, A., Hackmann, A., Steil, R., Clohessy, S., Wenninger, K., & Winter, H. (2002). The nature of intrusive memories after trauma: The warning signal hypothesis. *Behaviour Research and Therapy, 40*, 1021–1028.

Ehlers, A., Maercker, A., & Boos, A. (2000). PTSD following political imprisonment: The role of mental defeat, alienation, and permanent change. *Journal of Abnormal Psychology, 109*, 45–55.

Ehlers, A., & Steil, R. (1995). Maintenance of intrusive memories in posttraumatic stress disorder: A cognitive approach. *Behavioural and Cognitive Psychotherapy, 23*, 217–249.

Foa, E. B., Molnar, C., & Cashman, L. (1995). Change in rape narratives during exposure therapy for posttraumatic stress disorder. *Journal of Traumatic Stress, 8*, 675–690.

Foa, E. B., & Rothbaum, B. O. (1998). *Treating the trauma of rape. Cognitive-behavior therapy for PTSD*. New York: Guilford Press.

Foa, E. B., Steketee, G., & Rothbaum, B. O. (1989). Behavioral/cognitive conceptualisations of posttraumatic stress disorder. *Behavior Therapy, 20*, 155–176.

Gillespie, K., Duffy, M., Hackmann, A., & Clark, D. M. (2002). Community based cognitive therapy in the treatment of post-traumatic stress disorder following the Omagh bomb. *Behaviour Research and Therapy, 40*, 345–357.

Gray, M. T., & Lombardo, T. W. (2001). Complexity of trauma narratives as an index of fragmented memory in PTSD: A critical analysis. *Applied Cognitive Psychology, 15*, S171–S186.

Grey, N., Young, K., & Holmes, E. (2002). Cognitive restructuring within reliving: A treatment for peritraumatic emotional "hotspots" in posttraumatic stress disorder. *Behavioural and Cognitive Psychotherapy, 30*, 37–56.

Hackmann, A., Ehlers, A., Speckens, A., & Clark, D. M. (in press). Qualities and content of intrusive memories and their changes with treatment. *Journal of Traumatic Stress*.

Halligan, S. L., Michael, T., Clark, D. M., & Ehlers, A. (2003). Posttraumatic stress disorder following assault: The role of cognitive processing, trauma memory, and appraisals. *Journal of Consulting and Clinical Psychology, 71*, 419–431.

Harvey, A. G., & Bryant, R. A. (1999). A qualitative investigation of the organization of traumatic memories. *British Journal of Clinical Psychology, 38*, 401–405.

Hellawell, S. J., & Brewin, C. (2002). A comparison of flashbacks and ordinary autobiographical memories of trauma: Cognitive resources and behavioural observations. *Behaviour Research and Therapy*, *40*, 1143–1156.

Holman, E. A., & Silver, R. C. (1998). Getting "stuck" in the past: Temporal orientation and coping with trauma. *Journal of Personality and Social Psychology*, *74*, 1146–1163.

Holmes, E. A., Grey, N., & Young, K. A. D. (in press). Intrusive images and "hotspots" of trauma memories in posttraumatic stress disorder: An exploratory analysis of emotions and cognitive themes. *Journal of Behavior Therapy and Experimental Psychology*.

Joseph, S., Williams, R., & Yule, W. (1997). *Understanding post-traumatic stress. A psychosocial perspective on PTSD and treatment*. Chichester, UK: Wiley.

Keane, T. M., Zimmerling, R. T., & Caddell, J. M. (1985). A behavioral formulation of post-traumatic stress disorder in Vietnam veterans. *The Behavior Therapist*, *8*, 9–12.

Kilpatrick, D. G., & Veronen, L. J. (1983). Treatment of rape-related problems: Crisis intervention is not enough. In L. Cohen, W. Clairborn, & G. Specter (Eds.), *Crisis intervention* (pp. 165–185). New York: Human Services Press.

Koriat, A., Goldsmith, M., & Pansky, A. (2000). Toward a psychology of memory accuracy. *Annual Review of Psychology*, *51*, 481–537.

Koss, M. P., Figueredo, A. J., Bell, I., Tharan, M., & Tromp, S. (1996). Traumatic memory characteristics: A cross-validated mediational mode of response to rape among employed women. *Journal of Abnormal Psychology*, *105*, 421–432.

Markowitsch, H. J. (1995). Which brain regions are critically involved on the retrieval of old episodic memory? *Brain Research Reviews*, *21*, 117–127.

McNally, R. J. (2003). Psychological mechanisms in acute response to trauma. *Biological Psychiatry*, *53*, 779–786.

Mellman, T. A., & Davis, G. C. (1985). Combat-related flashbacks in posttraumatic stress disorder: Phenomenology and similarity to panic attacks. *Journal of Clinical Psychiatry*, *46*, 379–382.

Michael, T. (2000). *The nature of trauma memory and intrusive cognitions in posttraumatic stress disorder*. D.Phil. thesis, University of Oxford, UK.

Michael, T., & Ehlers, A. (2004). *Enhanced priming for trauma-related stimuli and PTSD symptoms: Two experimental investigations*. Manuscript in preparation.

Michael, T., Ehlers, A., & Halligan, S. L. (2004). *Enhanced priming for trauma-related material predicts posttraumatic stress disorder*. Manuscript submitted for publication.

Murray, J., Ehlers, A., & Mayou, R. A. (2002). Dissociation and posttraumatic stress disorder: Two prospective studies of road traffic accident victims. *British Journal of Psychiatry*, *180*, 363–368.

Porter, S., & Birt, A. R. (2001). Is traumatic memory special? A comparison of traumatic memory characteristics with memory for other emotional life experiences. *Applied Cognitive Psychology*, *15*, S101–S117.

Rachman, S. (1980). Emotional processing. *Behaviour Research and Therapy*, *18*, 51–60.

Resick, P. A., & Schnicke, M. K. (1993). *Cognitive processing therapy for rape victims*. Newbury Park, CA: Sage.

Reynolds, M., & Brewin, C. R. (1998). Intrusive cognitions, coping strategies and emotional responses in depression, post-traumatic stress disorder and a non-clinical population. *Behaviour Research and Therapy*, *36*, 135–147.

Reynolds, M., & Brewin, C. R. (1999). Intrusive memories in depression and posttraumatic stress disorder. *Behaviour Research and Therapy*, *37*, 201–215.

Schacter, D. L., Norman, K. A., & Koutstaal, W. (1997). The recovered memories debate: A cognitive neuroscience perspective. In M. A. Conway (Ed.), *Recovered memories and false memories* (pp. 63–99). Oxford: Oxford University Press.

Shalev, A. Y. (1992). Posttraumatic stress disorder among injured survivors of a terrorist attack. Predictive value of early intrusion and avoidance symptoms. *Journal of Nervous and Mental Disease*, *180*, 505–509.

Shobe, K. K., & Kihlstrom, J. F. (1997). Is traumatic memory special? *Current Directions in Psychological Science*, *6*, 70–74.

Steil, R., & Ehlers, A. (2000). Dysfunctional meaning of posttraumatic intrusions in chronic PTSD. *Behaviour Research and Therapy*, *38*, 537–558.

Tromp, A., Koss, M., Figueredo, A., & Tharan, M. (1995). Are rape memories different? A comparison of rape, other unpleasant, and pleasant memories among employed women. *Journal of Traumatic Stress*, *8*, 607–627.

Tulving, E. (2001). Episodic memory and common sense. In A. Baddeley, M. Conway, & J. Aggleton (Eds.), *Episodic memory. New directions in research* (pp. 269–288). Oxford: Oxford University Press.

Tulving, E. (2002). Episodic memory. *Annual Review of Psychology*, *53*, 1–25.

van der Kolk, B. A., & Fisler, R. (1995). Dissociation and the fragmentary nature of traumatic memories: Overview and exploratory study. *Journal of Traumatic Stress*, *8*, 505–525.

van der Kolk, B. A., & van der Hart, O. (1991). The intrusive past: The flexibility of memory and the engraving of trauma. *American Imago*, *48*, 425–454.

Van der Minnen, A. (2002). Changes in trauma narratives with exposure treatment *Journal of Traumatic Stress*, *15*, 255–258.

MEMORY, 2004, *12* (4), 416–427

Occurrence of imagery and its link with early memories in agoraphobia

Samantha J. Day

University College London, and The Traumatic Stress Clinic, Camden & Islington Mental Health and Social Trust, London, UK

Emily A. Holmes

The Traumatic Stress Clinic, Camden & Islington Mental Health and Social Trust, London, and MRC Cognition and Brain Sciences Unit, Cambridge, UK

Ann Hackmann

Department of Psychiatry, University of Oxford, and Institute of Psychiatry, London, UK

Recent cognitive models suggest that mental imagery can help us understand the maintenance of anxiety disorders (e.g., de Silva, 1986; Hackmann, Surawy, & Clark, 1998). However, imagery is relatively unexplored within agoraphobia. Such images are also thought to be useful in uncovering memories that occurred around the onset of a disorder (Hackmann, Clark, & McManus, 2000). A total of 20 patients with agoraphobia and 20 matched controls took part in this investigation. Participants described any recurrent images they experienced in agoraphobic situations, and also any associated memories. All patients with agoraphobia (but no control participants) reported having distinct recurrent images in "agoraphobic situations". Most images involved several sensory modalities and in the majority of cases appeared to be linked with unpleasant memories of events experienced many years previously. While these exploratory findings require replication, potential treatment implications are discussed.

The present study explores recurrent imagery and associated memories in participants with agoraphobia and matched controls. The imagery described is that which participants report experiencing in the type of situations that are anxiety provoking for people with agoraphobia. *DSM-IV* (American Psychiatric Association, *Diagnostic and Statistical Manual of Mental disorders,* 4th ed., 1994) defines agoraphobia as "anxiety about being in a place(s) or situation(s) from which escape might be difficult (or embarrassing) or in which help may not be available in the event of having a panic attack ... or panic-like symptoms (e.g., fear of the consequences of having a sudden attack of dizziness or ... diarrhoea)".

To our knowledge the occurrence and content of imagery in those with agoraphobia have not been explored, with the exception of one study investigating the perspective taken in images, which used people experiencing agoraphobic fears in a comparison group. Wells and Papageorgiou (1999) found that patients with social phobia and agoraphobia (but not blood injury phobia) reported taking an observer perspective while imagining a recent anxiety-provoking social situation. They speculated that this is because both groups have social evaluative concerns. Unlike people with social phobia, those with agoraphobia also seemed to maintain an observer perspective while imagining a non-social, non-

Correspondence should be addressed to Dr Emily A. Holmes, MRC Cognition and Brain Sciences Unit, 15 Chaucer Road, Cambridge CB2 2EF, UK. Email: emily.holmes@mrc-cbu.cam.ac.uk

Peter Scragg, Chris Barker, Pasco Fearon, and Agnes van Minnen provided helpful discussions and statistical advice. We would like to thank the clinical psychologists who helped to recruit participants for this study, especially John Cape and Peter Butcher.

DOI:10.1080/09658210444000034

anxiety-provoking situation. However, in this study participants rated perspective on a continuum between observer and field perspective, whereas clinical experience indicates that perspective may actively alternate between the two extremes. There are also other aspects of imagery in agoraphobia that would be interesting to explore. Recent studies have highlighted the importance of imagery in the maintenance and treatment of other anxiety disorders (Brewin & Holmes, 2003; Clark & Wells, 1995; de Silva, 1986; Hackmann et al., 2000; Hackmann et al., 1998; Holmes, Grey, & Young, in press; Wells & Hackmann, 1993). Such research includes social phobia, post-traumatic stress disorder (PTSD), and health anxiety, as well as insomnia (Harvey & Payne, 2002).

Overall, since research in imagery has positively influenced the development of treatment strategies in other anxiety disorders, we believe it is pertinent to investigate imagery in agoraphobia. For example, research within social phobia (Clark & Wells, 1995; Hackmann et al., 2000; Hirsch, Meynen, & Clark, 2004 this issue) suggests that anxiety (at least in part) is maintained by a distorted, negative image of one's public self, where the image of the self is seen from a perspective of an observer. This has guided successful treatment development using video feedback to update this image (e.g., Harvey, Clark, Ehlers, & Rapee, 2000). It has also been argued that exploring images is an effective way of uncovering underlying, problematic beliefs in social phobia (Hackmann et al., 2000) as well as health anxiety (Wells & Hackmann, 1993). Further, Hackmann et al. (2000) found that in 20 patients with social phobia all their reported recurrent images appeared to be linked to unpleasant early memories that tended to be clustered around the onset of the disorder. It would be useful to see whether these interesting findings extend to agoraphobia, and in addition, to use a non-clinical control group to examine whether or not they also report recurrent images in agoraphobic-type situations.

Recent conceptualisations of agoraphobia (e.g., Salkovskis & Hackmann, 1997) have highlighted the role of pre-existing beliefs and assumptions in the maintenance of the disorder. Reviews of the literature suggest that individuals with panic disorder who suffer from agoraphobic avoidance differ from those who do not in important ways. They may be more dependent and less self-sufficient, and they have a history of separation anxiety (for a review see Hackmann,

1998a). Bearing this in mind, consideration of the threat appraisal model (Clark, 1988; Salkovskis, 1988, 1991; Salkovskis, Clark, & Gelder, 1996) suggests that people with extensive agoraphobic avoidance may worry more about the perceived interpersonal "cost" of a mental or physical catastrophe, in addition to worrying about their perceived poor coping ability and the possible lack of rescue factors. It is predicted that if people with agoraphobia experience imagery reflecting such worries in threatening situations, this may influence their evaluation of danger, and their avoidance behaviour. Threatening situations would include typical "agoraphobic situations", such as being in a crowd or an enclosed space.

Horowitz (1970) defined imagery as mental contents that possess sensory qualities, as opposed to mental activity that is purely verbal and abstract. Images can include qualities from any sensory modality, such as vision, touch, hearing, taste, and smell. Visual components are thought to be the most common in anxiety disorders (Hackmann, 1998b). Cognitive behavioural therapy in general has largely focused on the use of patients' verbal contents of consciousness rather than imagery. However Beck (1976) originally proposed that distorted appraisals can be accessed via images and memories as well as verbal thoughts. Further, using only a linguistic mode in therapy could limit the depth of meaning accessed (e.g., Hackmann, 1998b; Sheikh & Jordan, 1983).

There has recently been a resurgence of treatments using imagery (e.g., Arntz & Weertman, 1999; Rusch, Grunert, Mendelsohn, & Smucker, 2000). Intriguingly, Rusch et al. (2000) carried out a treatment trial of imagery rescripting for patients with PTSD using only one session. The trial resulted in a marked decrease in the frequency and emotional impact of the image. We speculate that it might therefore be interesting to examine symptom levels 1 week after our imagery interview to assess if there might be any impact.

This exploratory study had three main aims. First, we aimed to investigate whether people with agoraphobia report experiencing recurrent imagery in agoraphobic situations, such as crowded or enclosed places. If imagery is reported, its characteristics, including sensory modalities and the perspective taken in the image, will be explored. Reports concerning recurrent imagery in people with agoraphobia will be compared with those from a sample of matched, non-clinical, control participants. Second, we aimed to investigate whether participants consider their images to be associated with a particular autobiographical memory. Third, we planned to assess agoraphobic symptoms both at the initial interview and again after 1 week, to investigate any impact of the interview.

METHOD

Participants

A total of 20 patients with agoraphobia (15 women and 5 men) and 20 non-clinical controls, matched for age and gender, participated. Participants with agoraphobia had been referred for therapy to one of four outpatient psychology departments in a large city. All were on a psychology waiting list for treatment of their agoraphobia. The diagnosis of agoraphobia had been made by the health professional responsible for their care. This diagnosis was checked against *DSM-IV* (APA, 1994) criteria during the interview for the current study, indicating that all patients had symptoms consistent with criteria for panic disorder with agoraphobia. None met criteria for a diagnosis of agoraphobia without history of panic disorder. Two participants also fulfilled criteria for PTSD (although the index trauma reported was not that described later as

the "associated memory"), and one for obsessive-compulsive disorder. The anxiety and phobic avoidance in these three patients was judged as not being better accounted for by their co-morbid diagnoses. The mean age of participants with agoraphobia was 48.9 years (SD = 16.3). The reported mean age of onset of agoraphobia was 34.5 years (SD = 11.6). The control group comprised 20 people matched for age (M = 48.3 years, SD = 18.9) and gender (15 women and 5 men). They were contacted through a local hairdressing salon to facilitate comparability in terms of socio-economic status. There was no significant difference between groups for number of years in education, $t(28.2)$ = 1.15, p = .26; the mean in the agoraphobia group was 12.0 (SD = 2.7), and in the control group 13.5 (SD = 5.2).

Measures

Symptom questionnaires. All participants completed the following questionnaires at the time of the interview: the Beck Anxiety Inventory (BAI: Beck, Epstein, Brown, & Steer, 1988), the Beck Depression Inventory (BDI: Beck, Ward, Mendelsohn, Mock, & Erbaugh, 1961), the Fear Questionnaire (FQ: Marks & Mathews, 1979), and the Mobility Inventory for Agoraphobia (MIA: Chambless, Caputo, Jasin, Gracely, & Williams, 1985). Table 1 shows mean scores on each mea-

TABLE 1
Scores on questionnaires measuring anxiety, mood, and agoraphobic symptoms for the patient and control groups

Questionnaire	Participants with agoraphobia		Control participants		t	df	p
	M	SD	M	SD			
BAI	29.8	9.8	4.3	3.3	11.1	23.3	**
BDI	24.1	11.7	6.3	5.7	6.0	25.9	**
FQ total	69.5	19.6	14.4	7.8	11.7	38.0	**
FQ subscales:							
Agoraphobia avoidance	32.6	5.4	1.7	2.0	24.0	24.0	**
Blood-injury avoidance	16.3	9.1	6.2	4.7	4.4	28.6	**
Social avoidance	20.6	10.7	6.6	4.1	5.5	24.6	**
Anxiety and depression	24.5	8.0	9.0	5.9	6.9	38	**
Present severity of phobia	5.8	1.4	0.5	0.8	14.8	38	**
MIA subscales:							
Avoidance when accompanied	95.9	15.6	27.1	6.8	18.1	25.9	**
Avoidance when alone	111.4	13.6	29.9	9.1	22.3	38	**
Number of panic attacks in last week	1.3	1.8	0.1	0.3	2.8	20.1	*
Intensity of panic attacks	1.7	1.8	0.0	0.0	4.0	19.0	**

BAI = Beck Anxiety Inventory; BDI = Beck Depression Inventory; FQ = Fear Questionnaire; MIA = Mobility Inventory for Agoraphobia.
** = p < .001; * = p < .05

sure, which indicate that all patients and none of the controls were experiencing clinical levels of agoraphobic symptoms. If Levene's statistic was significant, homogeneity of variance was not assumed. A Bonferroni correction was administered on the items due to the number of *t*-tests carried out.

The imagery interview. The Imagery Interview Schedule (Hackmann et al., 2000) was modified for use in this study. In the modification, we included a preliminary relaxation situation, in order to familiarise all participants with discussing their mental imagery. A set of five typical agoraphobic situations was constructed from the Fear Questionnaire (Marks & Mathews, 1979) to use as example situations in which imagery may occur. An anagram task was used to provide a break between the imagery and the memory questions (MacLeod, Williams, & Bekerian, 1991). Administration of the imagery interview took approximately 30 minutes. Details are given in four sections below, for clarity.

Interview Section 1: Relaxation images. The participant was asked to close their eyes and imagine a pleasant situation on a beach. Participants were asked to describe sensory characteristics in order to familiarise them with the process of answering questions about mental imagery. Participants were also asked whether their predominant viewpoint in the image was one of three types: a field perspective (seeing out of their own eyes); an observer perspective (as if viewing themselves as an observer); or, unlike Wells and Papageorgiou (1999), also whether it alternated between these two positions.

Interview Section 2: Agoraphobic situation images. Participants at this stage in the interview had all confirmed that they understood what was meant by a mental image during the relaxation phase. They were then asked if they experienced any recurrent images (e.g. "fleeting pictures you might have experienced again and again") in typical agoraphobic situations, especially "in situations that make you anxious". If so, they were asked to describe the types of situation and associated images. Our standard interview procedure for both groups included the same questions and further prompts. However, we found that all participants with agoraphobia immediately described a situation that matched our typical agoraphobic situation criteria, and did not require further

prompts. All control participants required prompting for situations. They then chose their most fearful situation from the five typical agoraphobic situations, and were encouraged to generate an image from this.

Once the participant indicated they had an image in mind, they were asked to "close your eyes and recreate one of those images now, making it as vivid as possible, so that a film director might be able to recreate the scene" and to describe their image. They were then asked to confirm or not whether the image included each of five sensory modalities (visual, sounds, body sensations perceptions, taste, and smell representations). They were asked to rate what the viewpoint of their image was: field, observer, or alternating perspective, as above. They were also asked "what does this memory mean about you, others and the world?".

Interview Section 3: Associated memory. Participants were asked to endorse whether they could or could not recall a particular memory that seemed closely linked to the image, in terms of the sort of emotions, thoughts, and sensations reflected in the image. Participants were asked what age they were at the time the event in this memory was experienced. The participant then engaged in the anagram task for 5 minutes (MacLeod et al., 1991). After this break, participants were asked to evoke their memory (the memory they linked to the image) with their eyes closed as if it was happening now, and to describe it. Information was gained about the sensory characteristics, perspective, and qualitative features of the selected memory as in the Interview Section 2 above. They were also asked "what does this memory mean about you, others and the world?"

Interview Section 4: Link between memory and image. Participants were asked whether they had experienced anxiety in agoraphobic situations prior in time to the event described in their memory. They were also asked whether they thought the event in the memory impacted on their anxiety in agoraphobic situations currently.

Procedure

All participants were interviewed individually in their homes after giving their informed consent to the study. All participants completed all questionnaires and the full imagery interview, which took approximately 1 hour. The interview was recorded on audio-tape. Participants were then asked whether they would fill in another set of the same questionnaires 1 week after the interview, and all agreed. A stamped addressed envelope was provided for them to return the questionnaires to the researcher. After the session, all participants were carefully debriefed. They were given details of how to call the researcher if they wanted to speak further, although none did this. The sections of the audio-tapes of the interview in which each participant described their image, and associated memory were transcribed verbatim for subsequent analysis

Coding of transcripts

Two independent coders rated verbal transcriptions of the fear images and the associated memories on a 7-point emotional valence rating scale which was specified at each level, ranging from –3 (description is extremely negative and indicates actual catastrophe) to +3 (description is extremely positive and indicates no catastrophe). For further detail for each level, see Hackmann et al. (2000). The themes from the transcripts of the images and associated memories were analysed using a content analysis approach (Smith, 2000). This is discussed in further detail elsewhere (Day & Holmes, 2004).

RESULTS

Frequency of recurrent images in agoraphobic situations

All 20 of the participants with agoraphobia reported experiencing recurrent, distressing imagery in agoraphobic situations. All participants with agoraphobia spontaneously gave appropriate examples of agoraphobic situations and associated images. All of the control participants required prompting, that is, chose one of the pre-selected agoraphobic situations to generate an image of how it might feel to be in that situation. None of the control group reported experiencing recurrent images in agoraphobic situations.

Characteristics of images reported by participants

The sensory modalities reported as present or absent in the relaxation scenes and in the agoraphobia situation images are shown in Table 2. The sensory modality data are first compared between groups, and then also within groups. For the agoraphobic situation images, all participants in both patient and control groups reported that their images included representation in the visual modality. In the agoraphobic situation image, all

TABLE 2
For the relaxation and agoraphobic situation images, the percentage of participants who endorse that the image is represented in various sensory modalities, in both agoraphobia and control groups

| | Recurrent image | | | | | | |
| | Participants with agoraphobia | | Control group | | | | |
Sensory modality	N	%	N	%	χ^2	df	p
Relaxation image							
Visual	20	100	20	100			
Body sensations	5	25	0	0	5.7	1	*
Sounds	14	70	16	80	5.3	1	.47
Touch	3	15	15	75	14.5	1	*
Taste/smell	12	60	17	85	3.1	1	.08
Agoraphobic situation image							
Visual	20	100	20	100			
Body sensations	20	100	17	85	14.0	1	.71
Sounds	9	45	16	80	5.2	1	*
Touch	4	20	8	40	1.9	1	.17
Taste/smell	1	5	9	45	8.5	1	*

* = p <.05

of the agoraphobic group (100%) and most of the control group (85%) endorsed body sensation perceptions, and there was no significant difference between groups. Further, for this image, the agoraphobic group reported significantly less sound and taste/smell representations than the controls. However, for the relaxation image there was a significant difference in report of body sensation and touch representations, with the patient group endorsing more body sensation and less touch representations than the control group. There were no significant differences for the other modalities (see Table 2).

Within groups, modality scores were compared in the relaxation situation and the agoraphobic situation using McNemar's Test. This indicated that in both groups body sensations were reported significantly more often in the agoraphobic situation than the relaxation situation (agoraphobia group, $p < .001$; control group, $p < .001$). Further, in both groups taste/smell representations were reported significantly less often in the agoraphobic situation than the relaxation situation (agoraphobia group, $p < .05$; control group, $p < .001$). No other comparisons were significant.

For the relaxation image, there was no significant difference in report of perspective taken between the two groups, $\chi^2(2, N = 40) = 1.7$, $p = .40$ (see Table 3). However, for their agoraphobic situation image, there was a significant difference between the two groups in reported image perspective, $\chi^2(2, N = 40) = 7.2$, $p < .05$, with a more frequent alternating perspective reported in the agoraphobic group. As shown in Table 3, partici-

pants with agoraphobia reported a predominantly alternating perspective in their agoraphobic situation image compared to a field perspective in their relaxation image. McNemar's Test indicates that this difference was significant ($p = .0002$) within the agoraphobic group. There was no significant difference between the equivalent images within the control group ($p = .39$). Further comparisons were non-significant.

Two independent coders rated verbal transcriptions of the fear images on a 7-point emotional valence rating scale which was specified at each level, ranging from –3 (description is extremely negative and indicates actual catastrophe) to +3 (description is extremely positive and indicates no catastrophe). Comparison of scores between raters showed full agreement. The mean emotional valence ratings score for the agoraphobic group was –2.25 ($SD = 0.85$) compared to –0.09 ($SD = 0.91$) for the control group. The emotional valence ratings of the recurrent images of the agoraphobic group indicated that they were coded as significantly more distressing, $t(38) = 4.8$, $p < .005$, than the images generated by the control group.

Report of memories associated with images

Within both groups, all participants identified a particular memory that was closely associated with their report of imagery in agoraphobic situations. The age of the participant at the time of event in their associated memory differed sig-

TABLE 3
Endorsement of the perspective taken in relaxation and agoraphobic situation images, by both patient and control groups

	Participants with agoraphobia (N = 20)	Control participants (N = 20)
Relaxation image		
Field	11	12
Observer	5	2
Alternating	4	6
Agoraphobic situation image		
Field	2	9
Observer	1	2
Alternating	17	9

Field perspective (looking out their own eyes); Observer perspective (seeing themselves as if an observer); Alternating (fluctuating between the two perspectives).

nificantly between the groups: $t(31.9) = 2.8$, $p <$ .05; agoraphobic group $M = 14.3$ years, $SD = 13.4$, control group $M = 30.0$ years, $SD = 21.5$. The type and frequency of events described in the memories reported as associated with images are shown in Table 4.

Interestingly, in the agoraphobic group, 35% spoke about a memory of an abusive event at home that they thought was closely associated with their agoraphobic imagery. Such events included abuse by a parent, being neglected by parents, a parent being drunk and frightening, being locked in a bedroom, and mental or physical victimisation by another family member. Additionally, 25% of the agoraphobic group reported a memory of the threat of, or actual, attack by a non-family member. The two participants diagnosed with PTSD did not report their index trauma as the "associated memory".

The two independent raters then rated the emotional valence of the transcripts of the described memories, using the same scale described above for the emotionality ratings of images. The mean emotional valence ratings for memories described by the agoraphobic group was -2.4 $(SD = 0.75)$ and -1.5 $(SD = 0.89)$ for the control group. The emotional valence of the agoraphobic memories was coded as significantly more distressing than the control group, $t(38) = 3.45$, $p < .005$. In all cases, data showed that only the three negative points of the scale and the midpoint of the scale were endorsed. Between raters, the allocation of these four points was in full accordance for all but one participant with agoraphobia, indicating very high inter-rater agreement.

Themes of imagery and associated memories

A content analysis approach (Smith, 2000) was used to analyse the themes in the transcripts (see Day & Holmes, 2004). In summary, significant themes included mental or physical catastrophe, disorientation, amplified awareness of sensory perception, fear, social humiliation, intimidation, and lack of protection by others.

Examples of imagery and associated memories

The following examples illustrate the spontaneous imagery reported as experienced in agoraphobic situations, as described (verbatim) by people with agoraphobia, as well as associated memories. After describing the memory, participants were also asked, "what does this mean about you, others and the world?" and these responses are also included.

Participant 4:
Description of image experienced in agoraphobic situation: Stranded in a supermarket. Couldn't move. People around. Not being able to move. See faces, not moving like stuck monsters. High-pitched scream like white noise. Can hear the supermarket music and the sound of the fridges loud. Needing to stare at the food on the shelves and feeling I would fall over. Real people. Unable to surface. Feeling suffocated.
Response to question "What does this mean about you, others and the world?" I am fearful, powerless. Others are powerful. The world is split into

TABLE 4
The types of event reported in memories associated with images in agoraphobic situations, by participants in the agoraphobia and control group

| | Participants with agoraphobia | | Control participants | |
	N	*%*	*N*	*%*
Neglect/Abuse at home	7	35	0	0
Potential/or actual attack	5	25	3	15
Panic on public transport	3	15	2	10
Being stuck in an enclosed place	3	15	1	5
Near death experience	1	5	0	0
Being shown up in front of others	1	5	4	20
Shopping/being in a crowded place	0	0	6	35
Being lost as a child	0	0	3	15
Feeling lonely	0	0	1	5

those that are powerful and those who are powerless.

Associated memory: Age six or seven on a beach, I was in the sea. Feeling of drowning in the sea. Parents oblivious. Swallowing loads of water, feeling terror. Fear of not being able to get out. No one to help. Physical terror of swallowing salt water. Fear couldn't get out. I had to do it. Parents did not realise seriousness of situation.

Response to question "What does this mean about you, others and the world?" Was physically weak. I am not protected, helpless, weak. As a child (I) had to look after myself. No one there for me. Had to take control. People are not there to help. I have great difficulty asking for help. If they do not know you need it, can't give it. The world is only able to give help if it knows you need it.

Participant 5:

Description of image experienced in agoraphobic situation: On a tube train and it stops. Trying not to show fear, but being terrified. Looking at other people's shoes and feet. Having inner fear. Train stopping. Carriages closing in around. Seeing myself and how I look. Things closing in on me.

Response to question "What does this mean about you, others and the world?" I am pathetic, a coward, no need for it. Others have no feelings at all. The world is pretty shitty.

Associated memory: Age 22 working in construction. Lowered down into a tunnel four foot diameter to do some work. Called up and other people went for tea break. Just forgot about me in the tunnel, didn't think. I couldn't climb out, felt really afraid. Couldn't climb out. Really afraid for half an hour. Couldn't show my fear to anyone, would seem like weakness.

Response to question "What does this mean about you, others and the world?" I am fearful, get scared easily. People are fine, they don't mean harm. Didn't show malice. The world is things happen.

Participant report of the importance of the associated memory

A total of 75% of the agoraphobic group reported that they were not anxious in agoraphobic-type situations before experiencing the event that occurred in the memory. Significantly more participants in the agoraphobic group (75%) than the control group indicated that the experience in the memory impacted on their anxiety in agoraphobic situations (30%), $\chi^2(2, N = 40) = 10.0, p < .05$. After the structured interview, several of the participants in the agoraphobic group said that they were surprised that they had not thought about the image and the associated memory before the interview, since they felt it might be a significant factor in their fears. Examples include, "I think this was where my fear began. I will talk about it with my therapist" and "No wonder I am scared like this".

Follow-up symptom questionnaires 1 week after the interview

Follow-up questionnaires were sent to participants 1 week after the interview. All participants who did not return the questionnaires were contacted again by post, but without further questionnaire return. Data were obtained from 13 (65%) of the agoraphobic group and 11 (55%) of the control group. Symptom scores at interview and post-interview were compared on the six previously described questionnaires. To protect for multiple comparisons, the questionnaire data were first analysed using mixed model ANOVAs, with a grouping factor of condition, and a within-participants factor of time. Two significant interactions were found between time and condition for the "agoraphobic avoidance" subscale of the Fear Questionnaire, $F(1, 22) = 10.67, p = .004$, and the "Avoidance when accompanied" subscale of the Mobility Inventory for Agoraphobia, $F(1, 22) = 4.6, p = .044$. All other comparisons from the questionnaires were non-significant.

These interactions were analysed using repeated measures *t*-tests. These indicated that within the agoraphobic group there was a significant decrease over time for agoraphobic avoidance as measured by the Fear Questionnaire, $t(12) = 2.98, p = .011$. The mean score at time 1 was 33.0 ($SD = 5.1$) and at time 2 was 26.7 ($SD = 11.0$). There was also a non-significant trend towards a reduction in avoidance when accompanied by another person for the agoraphobic group over time on the Mobility Inventory for Agoraphobia, $t(12) = 2.1, p = .058$. The mean score at time 1 was 93.1 ($SD = 15.8$) and at time 2 was 82.5 ($SD = 24.0$). Examination of the control group showed a trend towards an increase in "agoraphobic avoidance" as measured by the Fear Questionnaire: $t(10) = 2.12, p = .06$, time 1 $M = 1.10, SD = 1.76$, time 2 $M = 2.64, SD = 2.9$. In the control group there was no change in "avoidance when accompanied by another person" on the Mobility Inventory for Agoraphobia: $t(10) = 0.87, p = .40$, time 1 $M = 25.8, SD = 8.8$, time 2 $M = 28.0, SD = 5.5$.

It is possible that the sample of 13 participants with agoraphobia who returned their questionnaires may have been different from the 7 who did not. The characteristics and questionnaire scores at time 1 of responders and non-responders were therefore compared using *t*-tests. This showed that within the agoraphobia group there was no difference in terms of age, gender, BAI, BDI, Fear Questionnaire and its individual subscales, or the Mobility Inventory for Agoraphobia and its individual subscales, largest $t(17) = 1.36$. There were no significant differences within the control group on any of the above measures, largest $t(18) = 1.58$, except age. The mean age of responders in the control group was 36.1 ($SD = 11.8$) and non-responders 63.3 ($SD = 14.6$), $t(18) = 4.63$, $p < .001$. This indicates that overall responders and non-responders were similar at the time of the first interview, with the one exception of age within the control group.

DISCUSSION

To summarise, the key findings from this study were that all participants with agoraphobia, but no control participants, reported experiencing distressing, recurrent imagery in agoraphobic situations. This imagery in the agoraphobia group was reported as being associated with unpleasant memories of particular events. The experience described in these memories was recalled as occurring in adolescence, approximately 35 years ago. In participants with agoraphobia, the reported agoraphobic situation images were represented in several sensory modalities, not just the visual modality. Further, compared to a relaxation image, they were reported as being viewed from a perspective that alternated between field and observer viewpoints. Independent coders rated descriptions of both the agoraphobic situation images and their associated memories descriptions, as more distressing than those described by the control groups. Finally, there appeared to be some decrease in agoraphobic avoidance as measured by the Fear Questionnaire (Marks & Mathews, 1979) 1 week after administration of the imagery interview.

The findings of the present study extend the results of Hackmann et al.'s (2000) pioneering study of imagery in social phobia, to imagery in people with agoraphobia. In both these patient groups, all participants reported experiencing recurrent images in either social or agoraphobic situations respectively. Hackmann et al. (2000) reported that 96% of their social phobia sample reported an associated memory with their recurrent image. All the patients in the current study reported that they associated a particular memory with their agoraphobic image, interestingly one that typically came from adolescence. Similarly, Wells and Hackmann (1993) argued that for people with health anxiety, "in most instances" an early aversive experience was said to be linked to patients' imagery. In our study, a high proportion of the agoraphobic participants (75%) reported that they did not fear agoraphobic situations before the time of the recalled memory, and most (75%) reported that the event in the memory currently had an impact on their agoraphobic anxiety.

In the current study, participants in both the agoraphobia and control group reported that their images were represented in several sensory modalities, not just visual. This implies that any clinical work concerning imagery in agoraphobia should explore imagery multi-modally. It should be noted that an interpretation of the comparisons of images in the agoraphobia situation *between* groups must be made tentatively, since all participants with agoraphobia described spontaneous imagery, whereas all those in the control group constructed imagery deliberately in response to prompts. While comparisons of spontaneously occurring images with deliberately generated images should be treated with caution, it was felt that having a control group to compare characteristics of the imagery was of some interest, particularly as several clinical studies have not made comparisons with imagery in non-clinical samples. Whether there are differences between spontaneous versus constructed imagery *per se* remains to be tested. It is our impression that the participants with agoraphobia seemed able to spontaneously "flashback" to their images without using scripts, whereas no one in the control group was readily able to generate agoraphobic situation imagery without the prompt of a script. Therefore, it would not have been appropriate to use scripts with the participants with agoraphobia, and not possible to explore spontaneous imagery in the control group.

Both groups reported a high frequency of both visual and body sensations perceptions in agoraphobic situation images. It appeared that in the agoraphobia situation image, participants with agoraphobia endorsed having less sound and taste/smell representations than the control group. For the same comparisons, there were no between-groups differences for the relaxation image. It is possible that visual and body sensations representations are the most salient for people with agoraphobia, as the body focuses on senses that may alert the individual to future potentially anxiety-provoking situations (cf. Ehlers, Hackmann, Steil, Clohessy, Wenninger, & Winter, 2002; Martin & Williams, 1990).

In relation to the perspective taken in agoraphobic situation images, the agoraphobic group were more likely to report viewing their imagery from an alternating perspective (i.e., fluctuating between a field and observer perspective) than the control group. The perspective reported by the agoraphobia group in the agoraphobic situation image (predominantly alternating) was significantly different from that taken in the relaxation situation (predominantly field perspective). The equivalent within-group difference was not found for the control group. This interesting finding could characterise a changing focus, from looking at the self from an observer point of view in the catastrophic situation (perhaps reflecting social evaluative concerns), to looking at the situation from a field perspective. More thorough investigation is indicated. The difference between these results and those of Wells and Papageorgiou (1999) may be because the previous study did not provide the response option of an alternating perspective.

The emotional valence ratings given by independent markers to descriptions of agoraphobic situation images were more negative in the agoraphobia group than in the control group. Perhaps this is a manifestation of the catastrophic appraisals of events made by people with anxiety states, which have been widely discussed (Beck, Laude, & Bohnert, 1974; Hibbert, 1984). Similarly, the memories associated with these images were also rated as more negative and catastrophic for the agoraphobia group. As illustrated in Table 4, the events described included very stressful, and even traumatic events (APA, 1994). It was interesting that these memories were reported as occurring approximately three decades prior to the interview, when the participants with agoraphobia were in their adolescence, and possibly constructing their sense of self and goals (Conway & Pleydell-Pearce, 2000).

The work of Conway and Pleydell-Pearce (2000) may aid our understanding of the current results in several ways. Consistent with the authors' account of autobiographical memory, the images reported by participants with agoraphobia appeared to concern extremely negative, self-defining moments when their personal "goals" were severely challenged. The associated images (i.e., sensory-episodic memories) were reported as being recalled involuntary and directly rather than being deliberately constructed (Conway, 2001). They may have been triggered by cues related to the original experience. Direct retrieval can have the effect of "hijacking" the individual's attention onto the image and away from other current tasks. This indicates that having intrusive images in agoraphobic situations would be very disruptive and might influence ongoing behaviour. The way in which these negative images are interpreted by what Conway calls the "working self" could be very destabilising. It would be interesting to investigate the nature of the recollective experience of recalling such images, that is, how much when experiencing them people felt they were actually happening "now". The current research suggests it may be useful to further elaborate our understanding of agoraphobia in terms of models of autobiographical memory such as that of Conway and Pleydell-Pearce (2000). It is also interesting to note that all the control participants also reported linked autobiographical memories in connection with their self-generated images. These memories appeared to be of less distressing and more recent events, nevertheless some of the same processes may be at work. It would also be of interest to further link issues in agoraphobia with our understanding of other psychological disorders in which memory may appear to cause distress (Conway & Holmes, in press; Holmes, in press; Holmes, Brewin, & Hennessy, 2004).

A perhaps surprising finding in the current study was that at 1 week after the interview, the agoraphobic avoidance in participants with agoraphobia, as measured by the Fear Questionnaire, had significantly reduced. However, this finding should be regarded cautiously since only 65% of participants returned their questionnaire. Nevertheless, it is noted that a comparison between responders and non-responders in this group indicated that there was no significant difference between their baseline measures, therefore the reduced sample may be considered representative. Therapy using imagery techniques provides some support that an imagery interview might plausibly result in symptom reduction. For example, Arntz and Weertman (1999) argue that by accessing fear imagery, an original memory that may have led to generalised rules and assumptions may be recalled. Focusing on this memory may lead to reappraisal of the incident, in terms of the event being an exception rather than a rule. In the current study, it could be speculated that the focus on the agoraphobic situation imagery plus the recall of an associated memory, may have led to spontaneous reappraisal of the memory's meaning. Rusch et al. (2000) argue that imagery rescripting can occur in one session. It is possible that the interview also provided exposure to an image that is usually avoided (Lang, 1977; 1979). Therefore, our tentative finding may be worthwhile exploring in future studies. Ideally, the imagery interview should be compared with another interview that does not explore imagery or memories. Further, the follow-up measures should be collected from the person's home, rather than relying on participants to mail the questionnaires, which may be a difficult task for people with agoraphobia.

The findings of this study suggest there may be an association between the content of agoraphobic situation images and report of past unpleasant memories. This supports the idea that sensory images may be associated with specific autobiographical episodes (Conway & Pleydell-Pearce, 2000). Clinically, this has implications for our understanding of the onset and maintenance of agoraphobia. To our knowledge, there is no published previous research that has examined occurrence of images in agoraphobia and related memories, or the possible impact of treatment addressing such imagery. Focusing on imagery may provide a way of accessing past memories that contain information about the unique meanings to that individual. This may be an efficient way of understanding cognitive maintaining factors in agoraphobia in therapy. It may be that some images represent past "traumatic" memories, as in PTSD, and thus have treatment implications (Ehlers & Clark, 2000; Foa & Kozak, 1986; Grey, Holmes & Brewin, 2001; Grey, Young, & Holmes, 2002). Exploring such images may allow more successful emotional processing (Rachman, 1980).

There are several limitations to the current study, as previously discussed, including the 65% return rate of follow-up questionnaires, and the comparison of agoraphobic situation imagery being confounded on a spontaneous versus induced dimension. It would also be helpful to use a fuller and standardised clinical interview for diagnostic purposes. This is an exploratory study, and the current results suggest that further research is warranted to replicate and explore these results. Perhaps our most striking finding from a cognitive therapy perspective, is that all participants with agoraphobia, but no control participants, reported experiencing distressing, recurrent imagery in agoraphobic situations.

REFERENCES

American Psychiatric Association (1994). *Diagnostic and statistical manual of mental disorders* (4th ed.). Washington, DC: American Psychiatric Association.

Arntz, A., & Weertman, A. (1999). Treatment of childhood memories: Theory and practice. *Behaviour Research and Therapy, 37,* 715–740.

Beck, A. T. (1976). *Cognitive therapy and emotional disorders.* New York: New American Library.

Beck, A. T., Epstein, N., Brown, G., & Steer, R. A. (1988). An inventory for measuring clinical anxiety: Psychometric properties. *Journal of Consulting and Clinical Psychology, 56,* 893–897.

Beck, A. T., Laude, R., & Bohnert, M. (1974). Ideational components of anxiety neurosis. *Archives of General Psychiatry, 31,* 319–325.

Beck, A. T., Ward, C. H., Mendelsohn, M., Mock, J., & Erbaugh, J. (1961). An inventory for measuring depression. *Archives of General Psychiatry, 4,* 561–571.

Brewin, C. R., & Holmes, E. A. (2003). Psychological theories of posttraumatic stress disorder. *Clinical Psychology Review, 23*(3), 339–376.

Chambless, D. L., Caputo, G. C., Jasin, S. E., Gracely, E. J., & Williams, C. (1985). The Mobility Inventory for Agoraphobia. *Behaviour Research and Therapy, 23,* 35–44.

Clark, D. M. (1988). A cognitive model of panic attacks. In S. Rachman & J. D. Maser (Eds.), *Panic: Psychological perspectives* (pp.71–89). Hillsdale, NJ: Lawrence Erlbaum Associates Inc.

Clark, D. M., & Wells, A. (1995). A cognitive model of social phobia. In R. Heimberg, M. Liebowitz, D. A. Hope, & F. R. Schneiser (Eds.), *Social phobia: Diagnosis, assessment and treatment.* New York: Guilford Press.

Conway, M. A. (2001). Sensory-perceptual episodic memory and its context: Autobiographical memory. *Philosophical Transactions of the Royal Society of London Series B-Biological Sciences, 356,* 1375–1384.

Conway, M. A., & Holmes, E. A. (in press). Autobiographical memory and the working self. In N. R. Braisby & A. R. H. Gellatly (Eds.), *Cognitive psychology.* Oxford: Oxford University Press.

Conway, M. A., & Pleydell-Pearce, C. W. (2000). The construction of autobiographical memories in the self-memory system. *Psychological Review, 107,* 261–288.

Day, S., & Holmes, E. A. (2004). *Themes in mental imagery and related memories in agoraphobia: A content analysis approach.* Manuscript in preparation.

de Silva, P. (1986). Obsessional-compulsive imagery. *Behaviour Research and Therapy, 24,* 333–350.

Ehlers, A., & Clark, D. M. (2000). A cognitive model of posttraumatic stress disorder. *Behaviour Research and Therapy*, *38*, 319–345.

Ehlers, A., Hackmann, A., Steil, R., Clohessy, S., Wenninger, K., & Winter, H. (2002). The nature of intrusive memories after trauma: The warning signal hypothesis. *Behaviour Research and Therapy*, *40*, 1021–1028.

Foa, E. B., & Kozak, M. J. (1986). Emotional processing of fear: Exposure to corrective information. *Psychological Bulletin*, *99*, 20–35.

Grey, N., Holmes, E., & Brewin, C. R. (2001). Peritraumatic emotional "hot spots" in memory. *Behavioural and Cognitive Psychotherapy*, *29*, 367–372.

Grey, N., Young, K., & Holmes, E. (2002). Cognitive restructuring within reliving: A treatment for peritraumatic emotional "hotspots" in posttraumatic stress disorder. *Behavioural and Cognitive Psychotherapy*, *30*, 37–56.

Hackmann, A. (1998a). Cognitive therapy in panic and agoraphobia: Working with complex cases. In N. Tarrier, A. Wells, & G. Haddock (Eds.), *Treating complex cases: The cognitive behavioural therapy approach*. Chichester, UK: Wiley & Sons Ltd.

Hackmann, A. (1998b). Working with images in clinical psychology. In P.M. Salkovskis (Ed.), *Comprehensive clinical psychology, Vol. 6. Adults: Clinical formulation and treatment*. Oxford: Pergamon/Elsevier Science Ltd.

Hackmann, A., Clark, D. M., & McManus, F. (2000). Recurrent images and early memories in social phobia. *Behaviour Research and Therapy*, *38*, 601–610

Hackmann, A., Surawy, C., & Clark, D. M. (1998). Seeing yourself through others' eyes: A study of spontaneously occurring images in social phobia. *Behavioural and Cognitive Psychotherapy*, *26*, 3–12.

Harvey, A. G., Clark, D. M., Ehlers, A., & Rapee, R. M. (2000). Social anxiety and self impression: Cognitive preparation enhances the beneficial effects of video feedback following a stressful social task. *Behaviour Research and Therapy*, *38*, 1183–1192.

Harvey, A. G., & Payne, S. (2002). The management of unwanted pre-sleep thoughts in insomnia: Distraction with imagery versus general distraction. *Behaviour Research and Therapy*, *40*, 267–277.

Hirsch, C., Meynen, T., & Clark, D.M. (2004). Negative self-imagery in social anxiety contaminates social situations. *Memory*, *12*, 496–506.

Hibbert, G. A. (1984). Ideational components of anxiety: Their origin and content. *British Journal of Psychiatry*, *144*, 618–624.

Holmes, E. A. (in press). Intrusive, emotional mental imagery and trauma: Experimental and clinical clues. *Imagination, Cognition and Personality*.

Holmes, E. A., Brewin, C. R., & Hennessy, R. G. (2004). Trauma films, information processing, and intrusive memory development. *Journal of Experimental Psychology: General*, *133*, 3–22.

Holmes, E. A., Grey, N., & Young, K. A. D. (in press). Intrusive images and "hotspots" of trauma memories in posttraumatic stress disorder: An explora-tory investigation of emotions and cognitive themes. *Journal of Behavior Therapy and Experimental Psychiatry*.

Horowitz, M. J. (1970). *Image formation and cognition*. New York: Appleton-Century-Crofts.

Lang, P. J. (1977). Imagery in therapy: An information processing analysis of fear. *Behavior Therapy*, *8*, 862–886.

Lang, P. J. (1979). A bio-informational theory of emotional imagery. *Psychophysiology*, *16*, 495–512.

Martin, M., & Williams, R. (1990). Imagery and emotion: Clinical and experimental approaches. In P. Hampson, P. J. Marks, F. David, & J. T. E. Richardson (Eds.), *Imagery: Current developments*. Florence, KY: Taylor & Francis/Routledge.

MacLeod, A. K., Williams, J. M., & Bekerian, D. A. (1991). Worry is reasonable: The role of explanations in pessimism about future personal events. *Journal of Abnormal Psychology*, *100*(4), 478–486.

Marks, I. M., & Mathews, A. M. (1979). Brief standard self-rating for phobic patients. *Behaviour Research and Therapy*, *17*, 263–267.

Rachman, S. (1980). Emotional processing. *Behaviour, Research and Therapy*, *18*, 51–60.

Rusch, M. D., Grunert, B. K., Mendelsohn, R. A., & Smucker, M. R. (2000). Imagery rescripting for recurrent, distressing images. *Cognitive and Behavioral Practice*, *7*, 173–182.

Salkovskis, P. M. (1988). Phenomenology, assessment and the cognitive model of panic. In S. J. Rachman & J. Maser (Eds.), *Panic: Psychological perspectives*. Hillsdale, NJ: Lawrence Erlbaum Associates Inc.

Salkovskis, P. M. (1991). The importance of behaviour in the maintenance of panic and anxiety: A cognitive account. *Behavioural Psychotherapy*, *19*, 6–19.

Salkovskis, P. M., Clark, D. M., & Gelder, M. G. (1996). Cognition–behaviour links in the persistence of panic. *Behaviour Research and Therapy*, *34*, 453–458.

Salkovskis, P., & Hackmann, A. (1997). Agoraphobia. In G. C. L. Davey (Ed.), *Phobias: A handbook of theory, research and treatment*. Chichester, UK: John Wiley & Sons Ltd.

Sheikh, A. A., & Jordan, C. S. (1983). Clinical uses of mental imagery. In A. A. Sheikh (Ed.), *Imagery: Current theory, research and application*. New York: John Wiley & Sons.

Smith, C. P. (2000). Content analysis and narrative analysis. In H. T. Reis & C. M. Judd (Eds.), *Handbook of research methods in social and personality psychology*. Cambridge: Cambridge University Press.

Wells, A., & Hackmann, A. (1993). Imagery and core beliefs in health anxiety: Content and origins. *Behavioural and Cognitive Psychotherapy*, *21*, 265–273.

Wells, A., & Papageorgiou, C. (1999). The observer perspective: Biased images in social phobia, agoraphobia and blood-injury phobia. *Behaviour Research and Therapy*, *37*, 653–658.

MEMORY, 2004, 12 (4), 428–436

Spontaneously occurring images and early memories in people with body dysmorphic disorder

Selen Osman and Myra Cooper

University of Oxford, Warneford Hospital, Oxford, UK

Ann Hackmann

University of Oxford, and Institute of Psychiatry, London, UK

David Veale

University of London, UK

A semi-structured interview assessing the presence and characteristics of spontaneous appearance-related images was designed and administered. A total of 18 patients with body dysmorphic disorder (BDD) and 18 normal controls took part. The BDD patients were found to have spontaneously occurring appearance-related images that were significantly more negative, recurrent, and viewed from an observer perspective than control participants. These images were more vivid and detailed and typically involved visual and organic (internal body) sensations. The study also found that BDD images were linked to early stressful memories, and that images were more likely than verbal thoughts to be linked to these memories. Implications for theory and clinical practice are discussed.

Horowitz (1970) defined images as contents of consciousness that possess sensory qualities, as opposed to those that are purely verbal or abstract. While the visual modality is most prominently represented within mental imagery, images can, and often do, have qualities associated with any of the senses. In addition to this, images can also be divided into different types and categories. They may occur spontaneously, be deliberately generated, transformed, or suppressed. They may reflect past, present, or future perspectives and may be literal or symbolic. Compared to verbal thoughts, images may sometimes provide direct access to a holistic network of beliefs underlying emotional responses that may be difficult to identify through questioning alone (Hackmann, 1998).

There is also evidence to suggest that an important relationship exists between images and autobiographical memories. For example, the presence of mental imagery has been found to be a general predictor of memory specificity (Williams, Healy, & Ellis, 1999). Intrusive memories involving recall of event specific knowledge (ESK) (Conway & Pleydell-Pearce, 2000) are core symptoms of post-traumatic stress disorder (PTSD; American Psychiatric Association, 1994). These often manifest as images. Cognitive theories of PTSD (e.g. Brewin, Dalgleish, & Joseph, 1996) typically include reference to imagery, and link it to autobiographical memory and emotional processing.

Research examining the nature and meaning of imagery in different psychological disorders, and links to early memories, has grown in recent years. For example, patients with social phobia (Hackmann, Surawy, & Clark, 1998) have been shown to report experiencing significantly more spon-

Correspondence should be sent to Myra J. Cooper, Isis Education Centre, Warneford Hospital, Oxford, OX3 7JX, UK. Email: myra.cooper@hmc.ox.ac.uk

http://www.tandf.co.uk/journals/pp/09658211.html

DOI: 10.1080/09658210444000043

taneously occurring images in anxiety-provoking social situations than non-patient controls. These images are typically negative in content, involve seeing oneself from an observer perspective (i.e., from an external viewpoint), and are perceived as at least partially distorted when considered after the event (Hackmann et al., 1998).

The images of people with social phobia also appear to be recurrent and involve sensory components in a variety of modalities. For example, Hackmann, Clark, and McManus (2000) found that bodily sensations occurred as an aspect of imagery almost as often as visual sensations. Importantly, the reported recurrent spontaneous images were linked to particular memories of events that occurred close in time to the onset of the social phobia. Images and associated memories were well matched with regard to their sensory content in the various modalities. Similar findings have been reported in other disorders (e.g., health anxiety, Wells & Hackmann, 1993: agoraphobia, Day, Holmes, & Hackmann, 2004 this issue).

While research examining the nature and meaning of imagery in psychological disorders has grown in recent years, most of this work has focused on anxiety disorders, with little research exploring the existence of imagery in other psychological conditions. It might be hypothesised from a clinical perspective that mental imagery would be implicated in disorders of body image, which include the eating disorders (anorexia nervosa and bulimia nervosa), and a more specific disorder of body image concern, known as body dysmorphic disorder (BDD). This paper is concerned with examining the nature and content of imagery in BDD.

A key criterion for the diagnosis of BDD in DSM-IV (*Diagnostic and statistical manual of mental disorders*, American Psychiatric Association, 1994) is "a preoccupation with a defect in appearance ... the defect is either imagined, or, if a slight physical abnormality is present, the individual's concern is markedly excessive" (p. 466).

Cognitive behavioural models have been developed for the understanding and treatment of BDD (Veale et al., 1996). Veale (2002) subsequently hypothesised that BDD patients have idealised values about the importance of appearance and tend to view themselves as an aesthetic object. Clinical experience suggests that patients suffer from extreme self-consciousness, with negative images of themselves, viewed mainly from an observer perspective (similar to images in

social phobia). However, this has not been empirically investigated, nor has the possible input from memory.

The hypotheses in this study were as follows: (1) People with BDD will report having more spontaneously occurring images (that are negative and recurrent) when asked about their appearance, compared to control participants. (2) The sensory modality characteristics of BDD images, and the perspective from which they are observed, will differ to those of the control group. (3) Spontaneously occurring images in people with BDD will be linked to early memories and experiences. (4) Images in people with BDD are more likely to be associated with stressful early memories than verbal thoughts.

METHOD

Participants

A total of 18 patients with BDD (9 men and 9 women) and 18 control participants (9 men and 9 women) aged between 17 and 49 years took part in the study. The mean age in years was 27.50 (SD = 7.02) for the BDD group and 26.83 (SD = 6.67) for the control group. Patients with BDD were recruited from The Priory Hospital, North London, through their consultant psychiatrist. All gave their informed consent for the study. Those with concurrent dementia/organic brain disorder, schizophrenia, delusional disorder, substance misuse, and those with a primary diagnosis of an eating disorder were excluded.

Clinically there is some overlap in typical symptoms in BDD and eating disorders. Therefore, to confirm that participants had a primary diagnosis of BDD and did not have a co-morbid eating disorder, all were screened with the BDD and eating disorder modules of the Structured Clinical Interview for DSM-IV (SCID), (Spitzer, Williams, & Gibbons, 1996).

The control participants (non-clinical) were recruited by requesting volunteers from among hospital staff and colleagues.

Measures

The interviewer rated BDD patients on the Yale-Brown Obsessive Compulsive Scale (Y-BOCS) modified for BDD (Phillips, Hollander, Rasmussen, Arnowitz, DeCaria, & Goodman, 1997). This is a short 12-item semi-structured interview used to assess the severity of BDD symptoms. All participants also completed the Beck Depression Inventory-II (BDI-II; Beck, Steer, & Brown, 1996), Rosenberg Self-Esteem Inventory (RSE; Rosenberg, 1965), Fear of Negative Evaluation Scale (FNE; Watson & Friend, 1969), and The Body Consciousness Questionnaire (BCQ; Miller, Murphy & Buss, 1981).

Semi-structured interview

The semi-structured interview was adapted from Hackmann et al. (2000, 1998) and comprised two sections, one investigating spontaneously occurring imagery and one investigating thoughts. The interview was piloted on eight volunteers (two men and two women from each group). No modifications were made to the schedule and the pilot data were thus included in the main analysis.

Spontaneous imagery section of interview

In this section participants were asked to think about a recent time when they had felt really worried and anxious about their appearance. They were asked if they had *ever* experienced any spontaneous images (using Horowitz's 1970 definition) at such times. If no images were reported, participants were asked if they had ever experienced an impression of the way they thought they looked, or how others might see them at such times. This was to capture sensory impressions other than visual pictures, should the participants have understood this to be a distinction. They were also asked if any of the images or impressions were recurrent. Participants were asked to recreate and describe the content of one of these images or impressions. They were asked about each of the sensory modalities in the image/impression in the following order: visual ("*Can you see anything in your image?*"), auditory ("*Can you hear anything in the image?*"), kinaesthetic ("*Are you performing any acts in the image?*"), cutaneous ("*Do you notice any sensations of touch or pressure upon your skin, from an external source?*"; "*Are you touching anything in the image?*"), organic or internal bodily sensations ("*Do you notice any sensations inside your body?*"), gustatory ("*Do you notice any sensations of taste?*"), and olfactory ("*Do you notice any sensations of smell?*"). The characteristics of each modality were explored in detail (e.g., "*How vivid*

is the image/impression of yourself in your mind's eye?"), with participants rating their responses on a 101-point scale (e.g., 0 = not at all vivid, 100 = extremely vivid).

The perspective from which each participant observed their image/impression was rated on a 7-point scale. Scores ranged from +3 (observer perspective: seeing myself completely from an external viewpoint, as if from another person's vantage point) to −3 (observing myself completely through my own eyes, as if looking in a mirror). This scale contrasted the observer perspective not with the field perspective (as in Wells, Ahmad, & Clark, 1998), but with a variant of the field perspective, in which the subject is viewing their self through their own eyes, as if in a mirror. This was because pilot work suggested that many control subjects described their image in this way. A 7-point scale was also used (by participant and interviewer independently) to rate the emotional tone of the image/impression from −3 (extremely negative) to +3 (extremely positive).

Participants were then asked when in their life they had first experienced the sensations, thoughts, and feelings they had in the image/impression, and if there was a particular memory that seemed closely linked to it. They were asked to evoke a relevant memory, which was then explored, as with the image, in terms of its content and sensory qualities. They also rated the extent to which the memory resembled the image in terms of its sensory qualities, emotional significance, and interpersonal meaning. Again, 101-point scales were used for these ratings (e.g., 0 = not at all similar, 100 = extremely similar).

Verbal thoughts section of interview

In this section participants' appearance-related thoughts were explored in the same way as relevant aspects of their images.

Procedure

Participants were interviewed individually by the first author (SO). The semi-structured interview took between 45 and 120 minutes and the two sections were administered in counterbalanced order. All interviews were audio taped with participants' permission. Four participants from each group agreed to repeat the interview for test–retest purposes. All repeat interviews took place within 4 weeks of initial administration.

RESULTS

Analysis for normality (Kolmogorov-Smirnov Test) and equality of variance (Levene's Test for Equality of Variance) was carried out on the data. Parametric tests (e.g., independent t-test) were used where the assumptions for such testing were met. In all other cases, non-parametric equivalents were employed to assess between group differences (e.g., Mann-Whitney Test, Chi-square Test, Fisher's Exact Test) and within group differences (Wilcoxon Signed Ranks Test).

Descriptive data

Demographic data. The median number of years in full time education for each group, and inter-quartile ranges (IQR) were 14.00 (IQR = 12.00–15.00) and 15.00 (IQR = 13.75–16.00) respectively. There were no significant between-group differences for age ($t = 0.29$, $df = 34$, $p = .77$) or years in education ($U = 117.00$, $p = .16$).

Clinical characteristics. The mean age of onset of BDD was 14.50 years ($SD = 7.68$) and mean length of time in treatment was 7.92 months ($SD = 9.62$). For women, typical features of concern were their skin, eyes, hair, teeth, and genitalia. For the men, eyes, hair, and genitalia were also common concerns, as well as their nose and head size. On the Y-BOCS modified for BDD, the patients had a mean score of 34.06 ($SD = 8.28$), indicating that they had relatively severe symptoms. Medians (and IQR) for the self-report questionnaires for both groups are presented in Table 1.

According to questionnaire scores the BDD patients were more depressed (BDI-II: $U = 8.00$, $p < .001$), had lower self-esteem (RSE: $U = 4.50$, $p < .001$), and had higher fear of negative evaluation by others (FNE: $U = 24.00$, $p < .001$) than the control participants. Participants in the BDD group were also more conscious of their internal body sensations (BCQ private body consciousness: $U = 66.50$, $p = .002$) and external appearance (BCQ public body consciousness: $U = 55.00$, $p = .001$). No significant between-groups difference was found on the BCQ body competence sub-scale (BCQ body competence: $U = 132.00$, $p = .36$).

Reliability of the semi-structured interview

Test–retest reliability. Test–retest reliability was assessed (for the participants who repeated the interview) item-by-item using the Wilcoxon Signed Ranks Test. No significant between-group differences for the images/impressions were observed at retest for any of the sensory modalities.

Frequency of spontaneous images/ sensory impressions

All of the BDD patients reported experiencing either spontaneous images ($n = 17$, 94%) or other sensory impressions ($n = 1$, 6%) when worried or anxious about their appearance. Of the control participants, 15 (83%) reported either spontaneous images ($n = 6$, 33%) or sensory impressions ($n = 9$, 50%). Images and sensory impressions were collapsed into one category and are reported as images/impressions for the remainder of the analyses. There was no difference between the

TABLE 1
Medians (and IQR) for BDD and control participants on the self-report measures

Scale	BDD group (n = 18)	Control group (n = 18)
BDI-II	30.50 (16.50–46.25)	2.50 (0–6.25)
RSE	30.00 (28.00–36.00)	15.50 (11.00–19.50)
FNE	28.50 (26.75–30.00)	14.50 (7.75–19.50)
BCQ subscales		
Private body consciousness	16.00 (11.75–18.00)	9.00 (7.75–12.00)
Public body consciousness	20.00 (15.50–22.00)	12.00 (10.50–14.25)
Body competence	8.00 (6.75–9.00)	6.50 (6.00–10.00)

BDI-II = Beck Depression Inventory-II; RSE = Rosenberg Self-Esteem Inventory; FNE = Fear of Negative Evaluation Scale; BCQ = Body Consciousness Questionnaire.

patients and controls in reported frequency of spontaneous images/impressions (Fisher's Exact Test, $p = .11$).

Characteristics of spontaneous images/impressions

Of those experiencing spontaneous images/impressions, 17 (94%) in the patient group and 7 (46%) in the control group reported these to be recurrent. The difference was significant (Fisher's Exact Test, $p = .002$).

Sensory modality characteristics

The median number of modalities reported for the images/impressions was 2.00 (IQR = 1.00–2.00) for the patient group and 1.00 (IQR = 1.00–2.00) for the control group. This difference was significant ($U = 98.50$, $p = .04$).

The visual modality was the most commonly reported sensory modality for both patients and controls, followed by the organic modality. The latter consisted of feelings of anxiety, such as tingling sensations in the body part of concern and a feeling of butterflies in the stomach. No participants reported gustatory or olfactory sensations.

Differences between groups in imagery characteristics

The BDD group reported images/impressions that were visually more vivid ($U = 0.00$, $p < .001$), brighter ($U = 42.50$, $p = .02$), more detailed ($U = 32.50$, $p = .004$), and involved facial and bodily features that took up a greater proportion of the whole image ($U = 39.50$, $p = .01$) than control participants. The BDD images/impressions also involved organic sensations that were more vivid ($U = 6.00$, $p = .002$) and intense ($U = 8.50$, $p = .005$). Median scores (and IQR) for both groups can be seen in Table 2.

The observer/mirror perspective

The median ratings for perspective of the images/impressions were 3.00 (viewing myself completely from an external viewpoint, as if through the eyes of another, IQR = 3.00 to 3.00) for the BDD group and −3.00 (viewing myself completely from my own eyes, as if in a mirror, IQR = −3.00 to −3.00) for the control group. It is notable that the scale could have been collapsed, as participants used it as a categorical measure rather than a continuum, utilising only extreme ends of the scale. All BDD participants saw themselves from an observer perspective, while all control participants reported the mirror perspective.

Emotional tone of the images/impressions

The median participant ratings of the emotional tone of their images/impressions were −3.00 (IQR = −3.00 to −2.75) for the patient group and −1.00 (IQR = −1.00 to −1.00) for the control group. BDD patients' ratings were significantly more negative ($U = 28.50$, $p < .001$) than the control groups' ratings.

TABLE 2
Medians (and IQR) of sub-modalities for the BDD and control groups

Characteristics	BDD group (n = 15, 83%)	Control group (n = 12, 80%)	Significance level
Visual			
Vividness	90.00 (85.00–100.00)	10.00 (7.50–17.50)	****
Brightness	60.00 (40.00–70.00)	35.00 (10.00–50.00)	*
Detail	90.00 (60.00–100.00)	60.00 (12.50–68.75)	***
Proportion of whole image	80.00 (70.00–95.00)	50.00 (40.00–60.00)	*
	(n = 13, 72%)	(n = 5, 33%)	
Organic (internal sensations)			
Vividness	90.00 (52.50–95.00)	12.50 (8.75–51.25)	***
Intensity	90.00 (55.00–100.00)	37.50 (17.50–56.25)	*

$*p < .05$, $**p < .01$, $***p < .005$, $****p < .001$.

Characteristics of early memories associated with images/impressions

Of the 18 BDD patients who reported spontaneous images/impressions, 15 (88%) reported that they were associated with a particular stressful memory. The median age in years associated with the event that occurred in the memory was 11.50 (IQR = 10.00–21.50). Typical themes included: being teased and bullied at school (e.g. "*I was 10 years old and never got on with this boy in school. I remember one day asking him why he didn't like me and he said 'it's because you're ugly'.*") and self-consciousness about appearance changes during adolescence (e.g. "*I was very tall for my age and I remember queuing up in the playground after break time one day and seeing my reflection in the hall window. My whole face and body seemed out of proportion and I was about two heads taller than everyone else.*"). Inspection of the themes suggested that all the early memories could be placed in one (or both) of these two categories.

Of the 15 control participants who reported spontaneous images/impressions, only 2 (13%) reported these to be closely linked to a particular memory. The median age in which the memory occurred was 13.00 (IQR = 10.50–5.50). Significantly more BDD patients reported a particular memory associated with their images, $x^2(1)$ = 14.07, $p < .001$, than control participants.

Table 3 illustrates the number (and percentage) of BDD patients reporting each sensory modality represented within the associated early memories/experiences. One patient did not wish to discuss their memory. The characteristics of the early memories reported thus relate to the remaining 14 patients. For ease of comparison, the relevant data for images/impressions are also reproduced in this table.

TABLE 3
Number (and percentage) of BDD patients reporting sensory modalities within their images and associated memories

Modality	Images (n = 18)	Early memory (N = 14)
Visual	15 (83%)	14 (100%)
Organic (internal)	13 (72%)	12 (85%)
Auditory	1 (6%)	8 (57%)
Kinaesthetic	1 (6%)	6 (43%)
Cutaneous	1 (6%)	5 (36%)
Gustatory	0	0
Olfactory	0	0

The median number (and IQR) of modalities reported for the BDD group early memories was 2.50 (IQR = 0.75–4.00). As for images/impressions, the visual modality was the most frequently reported sensory modality, followed by the organic sensation modality. These memories were also mainly viewed from an observer perspective (median = 3.00, IQR = 2.00–3.00). Again, no patients reported the presence of gustatory or olfactory sensations. There was no difference between the median number of modalities reported in the BDD groups' spontaneous images/impressions and early memories (Z = −1.31, p = .19).

Mean sensory similarity reported between the spontaneous image/impressions and the associated memories was 60%, mean emotional similarity was 65%, and mean interpersonal similarity was 71%. Inspection of the data suggested that there was generally a close match between reported modalities, i.e., patients who experienced a particular modality in their images/impressions were also likely to experience that modality in the associated memory.

Characteristics of early memories accessed through verbal thoughts

A total of 11 BDD participants (61%) and 2 control participants (11%) reported early memories associated with thoughts. This difference was significant, $x^2(1)$ = 6.48, p = .04. The median age of the participants within the memories reported by the BDD participants was 15.00 years (IQR = 10.00–22.50). This was not significantly higher than the median age (11.50, IQR = 10–21.50) in the reported early memories associated with images/impressions (Z = −1.65, p = .86).

Finally, the images/impressions of the BDD participants were more likely than thoughts to be linked to stressful early memories, $x^2(1)$ = 3.74, p = .05.

DISCUSSION

In line with the hypotheses, BDD patients were found to have significantly more spontaneously occurring appearance-related images/impressions that were negative, recurrent, and viewed from an observer perspective, than control participants. These images/impressions were also more vivid and detailed, and typically involved a greater number of sensory modalities, the most common of which were visual and organic. Analysis revealed that these imagery characteristics could be reliably assessed over time. Given the suggestion that people with BDD tend to selectively attend to interoceptive information (Veale et al., 1996), and the notion that visual imagery is the most common type of imagery (Marks, 1973), the current finding that visual and organic sensations predominate is not surprising. Other modalities may predominate in other clinical populations (consistent with the content of the disorder and hypothesised psychological processes). For example, a recent study has indicated that the kinaesthetic and visual modalities were important in people anxious about spiders (Pratt, Cooper, & Hackmann, in press).

Thus, while the occurrence of spontaneously occurring appearance-related images/impressions was similar in both groups (implying that the presence of such imagery is in fact common in both clinical and non-clinical populations), the findings suggest that it is the quality of these images, rather than their presence, that differentiates individuals with, and those without, BDD.

The BDD patients reported more images/impressions viewed from an observer perspective than controls. Clark and Wells' (1995) model of social phobia suggests that observer perspective imagery is partly constructed from interoceptive information. In BDD as in social phobia, part of the input may also be from memory of previous stressful experiences, where individuals have come under scrutiny perceived as critical. Thus imagery may be unlikely to convey an accurate impression of actual appearance. Interestingly Veale and Riley (2001) note that negative images arise when BDD patients attempt to look in a mirror. They may avoid close scrutiny of the actual reflection, and thus images do not get updated. By contrast participants without BDD, who are presumably not over-worried about their appearance, can and do look in mirrors. Memories may be formed of times when they occasionally see images discrepant with their usual appearance.

Images/impressions in the BDD group were typically considered to be linked to early stressful memories. The age of BDD participants in these memories and the themes that emerged from them provide support for models that identify typical symptom onset in early adolescence (e.g., Rosen, Reiter, & Orosan, 1995; Veale et al., 1996).

The link between appearance-related images and early stressful experiences suggests that some people may develop negative self-images early on that may contribute to the development of BDD symptoms, and that fail to update. Three processes (suggested by Hackmann et al., 2000, in relation to social phobia) might help to explain this phenomenon in BDD. The first is an attentional bias, and relates to the increased self-focused attention observed in BDD patients when negative appearance-related images arise (e.g., in front of a mirror, Veale & Riley, 2001). Second, BDD patients frequently avoid situations in which negative evaluation (of appearance) by others is anticipated or, if such situations are not avoided, subtle in-situation safety behaviours (e.g., camouflage) are employed. Both of these processes may prevent patients from noticing information that might correct their distorted negative self-images. Third, when patients do receive positive feedback about their appearance, this usually occurs in verbal form and, as a consequence, may be poorly suited to modifying visual images (Hackmann et al., 2000). In addition to these processes, information from others may be discounted as untrue by BDD patients (e.g., "they are only saying it to be nice to me") or may not be considered of value, as some patients may be more concerned with failure to achieve their own aesthetic ideals, than the demands of others (Veale, Kinderman, Riley, & Lambrou, 2003).

The observer perspective found in the images of people with this disorder may be viewed as one possible consequence of maladaptive attentional processes. Thus, it is conceivable that treatment strategies aimed at the alleviation of dysfunctional self-focused attention might modify biased imagery in BDD. Wells and Papageorgiou (1998) demonstrated that exposure plus externally focused attention produced greater reductions in anxiety and negative beliefs than exposure alone in people with social phobia. Moreover, the attention condition resulted in a significant shift from the observer to the field perspective in imagery, while the exposure alone condition did not.

The current study provides some empirical evidence for the role of imagery in BDD, and thus some preliminary support for Veale's (2002) hypothesis that BDD patients view themselves as an aesthetic object with extreme self-consciousness. Existing cognitive models of BDD (Veale et al., 1996) have been revised to acknowledge the importance of these findings (Veale, 2004).

There are a number of limitations to this study. An important conceptual limitation relates to the vague and all-encompassing definitions of imagery within the literature. As a result of this, other sensory impressions were placed within the same category as images (as in the study reported by Hackmann et al., 1998). This raises some important empirical questions. Are "images" and "impressions" considered by participants to denote similar phenomena, or are they seen as qualitatively different, with the latter perhaps referring to a milder, less distressing type of imagery? Within the current study, participant numbers were too small to allow for a comparison between images and impressions, and as a result, this is an important conceptual issue that requires further investigation.

The current study relied on verbal self-reporting as the main method of data collection. However, describing one's cognitive processes and conveying them accurately is not always straightforward and can be especially problematic in the case of imagery (Kendall & Korgeski, 1979). Furthermore, while this study identified a link between spontaneously occurring imagery and early memories, it would be presumptuous to assume causality. More detailed qualitative and quantitative analysis is needed to clarify the possible mechanisms involved. Future research exploring imagery in BDD would benefit from a larger sample size, recruited from multiple settings. The psychometric properties of the semi-structured interview also require further investigation. At present, studies of imagery within the psychological disorders tend to be disorder-specific. However, the observed link between the observer perspective and social-evaluative concern in both social phobia and BDD suggests that it might be of greater benefit to focus on how images differ in relation to specific beliefs or themes. Finally, a more detailed examination of memories that are linked to appearance-related images might prove beneficial in informing current theories of BDD, as well as influencing clinical practice.

REFERENCES

American Psychiatric Association. (1994). *Diagnostic and statistical manual of mental disorder* (4th ed.). Washington, DC: American Psychiatric Association.

Beck, A. T., Steer, R. A., & Brown, K. (1996). *Beck Depression Inventory. Version 2.* San Antonio: The Psychological Corporation, Harcourt Brace & Co.

Brewin, C. R., Dalgleish, T., & Joseph, S. (1996). A dual representation theory of posttraumatic stress disorder. *Psychological Review, 103,* 670–686.

Clark, D. M., & Wells, A. (1995). A cognitive model of social phobia. In R. Heimburg & D. A. Liebowitz (Eds.), *Social phobia: Diagnosis, assessment, and treatment,* (pp. 69–93). New York: Guilford Press.

Conway, M. A., & Pleydell-Pearce, C. W. (2000). The construction of autobiographical memories in the self-memory system. *Psychological Review, 107*(2), 261–288.

Day, S. J., Holmes, E. A., & Hackmann, A. (2004). Occurrences of imagery and its link with early memories in agoraphobia. *Memory, 12,* 416–427.

Hackmann, A. (1998). Working with images in clinical psychology. In A. S. Bellack & M. Hersen (Eds), *Comprehensive Clinical Psychology, 6,* 301–317. Amsterdam: Elsevier.

Hackmann, A., Clark, D. M., & McManus, F. (2000). Recurrent images and early memories in social phobia. *Behaviour Research and Therapy, 38,* 601–610.

Hackmann, A., Surawy, C., & Clark, D. M. (1998). Seeing yourself through others eyes: A study of spontaneously occurring images in social phobia. *Behavioural and Cognitive Psychotherapy, 26,* 3–12.

Horowitz, M. J. (1970). *Image formation and cognition.* New York: Appleton Century Crofts.

Kendall, P. C., & Korgeski, G. P. (1979). Assessment and cognitive-behavioural interventions. *Cognitive Therapy and Research, 3,* 1–21.

Lang, P. J. (1985). The cognitive psychophysiology of emotion: Fear and anxiety. In A. H. Tuma & J. D. Maser (Eds.), *Anxiety and the anxiety disorders* (pp. 131–170). Hillsdale, NJ: Lawrence Erlbaum Associates Inc.

Marks, D. F. (1973). Visual imagery differences in the recall of pictures. *British Journal of Psychology, 64,* 17–24.

Miller, L. C., Murphy, R., & Buss, A. H. (1981). Consciousness of body: Private and public. *Journal of Personality and Social Psychology, 41,* 397–406.

Phillips, K. A., Hollander, E., Rasmussen, S. A., Arnowitz, B. R., DeCaria, C., & Goodman, W. K. (1997). A severity rating for body dysmorphic disorder: Development, reliability, and validity of a modified version of the Yale-Brown Obsessive Compulsive Scale. *Psychopharmacology Bulletin, 33,* 17–22.

Pratt, D., Cooper, M. J., & Hackmann, A. (in press). Imagery and its characteristics in people who are anxious about spiders. *Behavioural and Cognitive Psychotherapy.*

Rosen, J. C., Reiter, J., & Orosan, P. (1995). Cognitive-behavioural body image therapy for body dysmorphic disorder. *Journal of Consulting and Clinical Psychology, 63*(2), 263–269.

Rosenberg, M. (1965). *Society and adolescent self image.* Princeton NJ: Princeton University Press.

Spitzer, R., Williams, J., & Gibbons, M. (1996). *Instruction manual for the structured clinical interview for DSM-IV.* New York: New York State Psychiatric Institute.

Veale, D. (2002). Over-valued ideas: A conceptual analysis. *Behaviour Research and Therapy, 40,* 383–400.

Veale, D. (2004). Advances in a cognitive behavioural model of body dysmorphic disorder. *Body Image*, *1*, 113–125.

Veale, D., Gourney, K., Dryden, W., Boocock, A., Shah, F., Wilson, R. et al. (1996). Body dysmorphic disorder: A cognitive behavioural model and pilot randomised controlled trial. *Behaviour Research and Therapy*, *9*, 717–729.

Veale, D., Kinderman, P., Riley, S., & Lambrou, C. (2003). Self-discrepancy theory in body dysmorphic disorder. *British Journal of Clinical Psychology*, *42*, 157–169.

Veale, D., & Riley, S. (2001). Mirror, mirror on the wall, who is the ugliest of them all? The psychopathology of mirror gazing in body dysmorphic disorder. *Behaviour Research and Therapy*, *39*, 1381–1393.

Watson, D., & Friend, R. (1969). Measurement of social-evaluative anxiety. *Journal of Consulting and Clinical Psychology*, *33*(4), 448–457.

Wells, A., Clark, D. M., & Ahmad, S. (1998). How do I look with my mind's eye: Perspective taking in social phobic imagery. *Behaviour Research and Therapy*, *26*, 631–634.

Wells, A., & Hackmann, A. (1993). Imagery and core beliefs in health anxiety: Content and origins. *Behavioural and Cognitive Psychotherapy*, *21*, 265–273.

Wells, A., & Papageorgiou, C. (1998). Social phobia: Effects of external attention on anxiety, negative beliefs and perspective taking. *Behaviour Therapy*, *29*, 357–370.

Williams, J. M. G., Healy, H. G., & Ellis, N. C. (1999). The effects of imageability and predictability of cues in autobiographical memory. *Quarterly Journal of Experimental Psychology*, *52*A, 555–579.

MEMORY, 2004, *12* (4), 437–446

A preliminary study of autobiographical memory in remitted bipolar and unipolar depression and the role of imagery in the specificity of memory

Warren Mansell and Dominic Lam

Institute of Psychiatry, University of London, UK

Autobiographical memory was investigated in a sample of 19 individuals with remitted bipolar affective disorder and a community sample of 16 individuals with remitted unipolar depression who had similar low levels of current symptoms. Each participant was prompted to recall one positive memory and one negative memory, to rate it on several scales, and to describe it in detail. Relative to the remitted unipolar group, the remitted bipolar group reported more general than specific negative memories and more frequent recollections of the negative memory during their everyday life. Across the sample, 95% of all specific memories involved a mental image, whereas only 56% of all general memories involved a mental image, suggesting a role of imagery in the retrieval of a specific memory. Characteristic examples of memories are provided. These results are preliminary yet they suggest that patients with bipolar disorder in remission may show memory characteristics that are often associated with symptomatic unipolar depression.

Bipolar disorder, otherwise known as manic depression, affects up to 1–1.5% of the population (Bebbington & Ramana, 1995; Robins et al., 1984). It is a severe mental illness, which leads to high rates of hospitalisation and suicide (Goodwin & Jamison, 1990). People with this diagnosis experience episodes of clinical depression as well as episodes of mania, during which they show symptoms such as extremely elevated mood, pressure of speech, grandiose beliefs, and disinhibited and dangerous behaviour (Goodwin & Jamison, 1990). Most people with bipolar disorder experience multiple relapses. For example, Tohen, Waternaux, and Tsuang (1990) found a relapse rate of 90% over 4 years.

The current paper explores autobiographical memory in remitted bipolar disorder. Research on autobiographical memory in psychological disorders has developed from a number of perspectives. First, within PTSD and depression, many studies have identified distressing recurrent memories, characterised their themes, and linked them to past negative life events (e.g., Ehlers, Hackmann, Steil, Clohessy, Wenninger, & Winter, 2002; Reynolds & Brewin, 1999). For example, Reynolds and Brewin (1999) found that a group of patients with PTSD and a group of patients with unipolar depression without PTSD, were both characterised by their reports of vivid, distressing, and repetitive memories that they tried to avoid and suppress. Memories in PTSD typically related to assault, illness, or injury to the patient, whereas memories in unipolar depression related to family illness, injury, death, or interpersonal disputes. In a second strand of research within anxiety disorders and psychosis, autobiographical memories

Correspondence should be sent to Warren Mansell PhD, Department of Psychological Medicine, Psychological Treatments Box 096, Institute of Psychiatry, De Crespigny Park, Denmark Hill, London SE5 8AF, UK. Email: warren@mansellw.freeserve.co.uk; w.mansell@iop.kcl.ac.uk

Thank you to Emily Holmes for her valuable feedback in the early stages of the design of this study, and to Kim Wright for her frequent help with recruiting participants. Thank you to the participants who gave consent for the extracts of their memories to be reproduced here.

http://www.tandf.co.uk/journals/pp/09658211.html

DOI:10.1080/09658210444000052

have often been accessed by making links between spontaneous imagery in stressful situations and earlier childhood experiences (e.g., Hackmann, Clark, & McManus, 2000; Morrison et al., 2002; Wells & Hackmann, 1993). In these studies, the themes of the memories have been described in some detail. For example, memories in social phobia can include themes of intense criticism by an authority figure, or rejection or ridicule by peers (Hackmann et al., 2000).

Thus, it appears that vivid distressing recurrent memories are a characteristic of a range of psychological disorders including anxiety disorders, psychotic disorders, and unipolar depression. The themes of these memories appear to be closely associated with the specific concerns of the individuals with the disorder. Following on from these findings, it would be reasonable to propose that people with bipolar disorder may also report frequent recurrent memories involving their key concerns, although this appears not to have been tested. Cognitive accounts of bipolar disorder indicate that people with this diagnosis have particular concerns about striving to achieve challenging personal goals. A recent study has demonstrated that patients with remitted bipolar disorder report higher goal-attainment beliefs (e.g., "If I try hard enough I should be able to excel") than patients with remitted unipolar depression (Lam, Wright, & Smith, 2004b). Therefore, we might expect patients with remitted bipolar disorder also to report recurrent memories around these themes. Considering that people with bipolar disorder are vulnerable to extremes in high mood (mania) and low mood (depression), we predicted that they would have elevated frequencies of recollection of negative and positive autobiographical memories compared to remitted unipolar patients.

The larger proportion of research into autobiographical memory in psychopathology has explored whether autobiographical memory is accessed at a "specific" or a "general" level. Models of autobiographical memory (e.g., Conway & Pleydell-Pearce, 2000; Norman & Brobrow, 1979) suggest that memory is organised in a hierarchical fashion, with upper layers containing general information that are linked to the more specific and detailed lower layers. A general memory is either a summary of events that have occurred over an extended period of time (e.g., a period at secondary school) or a category of certain kinds of events (e.g., visits to the zoo). A specific memory is a description of an event that occurred at a particular time in a particular place (e.g., one's 21st birthday party). In the model by Conway and Pleydell-Pearce, the lower level of the hierarchy contains "event-specific knowledge" (ESK) that is rich in sensory-perceptual detail. For example, the ESK of a memory of a birthday party might contain information about the happy expressions on the faces of the guests, the sounds of music, and the taste of the birthday cake.

A task known as the Autobiographical Memory Test (AMT) was developed by Williams and Broadbent (1986) to explore autobiographical memory. In this task, participants are presented with negative and positive cue words and asked to retrieve a personal memory in response to the word. Empirical studies have demonstrated that the tendency to recall general rather than specific memories is a feature of certain psychological disorders such as unipolar depression (Williams & Dritschel, 1988; Williams & Scott, 1988) and posttraumatic stress disorder (McNally, Lasko, Macklin, & Pitman, 1995). It has been proposed that the advantage of remembering specific memories is that they can be re-experienced and thereby re-interpreted by the individual, and so help to generate suitable responses to similar future events (Williams, 1997). In line with this suggestion, research has shown that levels of specificity in autobiographical memory were highly correlated with problem-solving ability (Evans, Williams, O'Loughlin, & Howells, 1992). Also consistent with the negative effects of overgeneral memory on psychopathology, an overgeneral memory bias has been identified as an important vulnerability factor for recurrent depression (Brittlebank, Scott, Williams, & Ferrier, 1993).

Further research on autobiographical memory involves the question of whether specific memories are more likely to involve mental imagery. A study of a non-clinical sample indicates that the degree to which one can generate imagery from a cue word predicts whether that event can be recalled at the specific, rather than the general, level (Williams, Healy, & Ellis, 1999). This finding indicates that specific memories may be more likely to involve mental imagery than general memories. Consistent with this view, a brain-imaging study showed that the retrieval of a specific autobiographical memory in non-clinical participants is associated with a temporary but marked increase in the activation of the posterior regions, which are associated with sensory-perceptual processing and mental imagery (Conway, Pleydell-Pearce, & Whitecross, 2001).

As explained earlier, patients with a diagnosis of bipolar disorder often are vulnerable to frequent relapses of mania and depression. Therefore, we would predict that they would have a cognitive vulnerability in contrast to patients who have recovered from an episode of unipolar depression. A key cognitive vulnerability would be in the form of an overgeneral memory bias. To date, only one study has explored autobiographical memory in bipolar affective disorder. Scott, Stanton, Garland, and Ferrier (2000) found that patients in remission (i.e., not currently in a depressed or manic episode) recalled a higher ratio of general to specific memories than healthy controls. This suggests that even when not depressed or manic, people with bipolar affective disorder show the overgeneral memory bias that is normally associated with depression. In addition, the remitted bipolar patients showed poorer problem-solving ability and this was related to their tendency to recall overgeneral memories (as shown in unipolar depression by Evans et al., 1992). Scott et al. (2000) did not include a control group who had experienced depression but were currently well. Therefore it is possible that Scott et al.'s findings could be explained by the past experience of depression in the bipolar group rather than the recurrent experience of mania and depression that characterises bipolar disorder. In order to control for the past experience of depression, it would be appropriate to use a control group who had recovered from depression and had never experienced mania.

The current study used a remitted unipolar control group and tested three hypotheses:

1. We predicted that an overgeneral memory bias would not be an inevitable consequence of having experienced depression in the past, but that it would be a characteristic of the vulnerability of bipolar patients to recurrent episodes of mania and depression. Therefore, we predicted that people with bipolar affective disorder in remission would show an overgeneral memory bias relative to people who had experienced unipolar depression.

2. In an extension of Williams et al. (1999), we proposed that mental imagery would be associated with the recall of specific as opposed to general autobiographical memories.

3. We predicted that people with remitted bipolar affective disorder would experience frequent intrusions of past negative memories, as found in several other psychological disorders. We predicted that the frequent recollection of past negative memories during everyday life would not be an inevitable consequence of having experienced depression, and so the remitted unipolar group would report a significantly lower frequency of recollection of the negative memory relative to the remitted bipolar group. We also predicted that the bipolar group would experience more frequent recollections of positive memories, as may be expected from their experiences of periods with particularly elevated mood.

Finally, in an exploratory analysis, we investigated the properties of the negative and positive autobiographical memories in remitted bipolar affective disorder (in a similar, but not identical, way to Hackmann et al., 2000).

METHOD

Participants

Participants were 19 individuals with a diagnosis of Bipolar I Disorder, currently in remission, and 16 individuals with unipolar depression, currently in remission. As would be expected from clinical practice, the participants with remitted bipolar affective disorder had received their diagnosis from a psychiatrist, whereas the participants with a past episode of unipolar depression had received their diagnosis from either a psychiatrist or a general practitioner. The diagnosis was confirmed at the end of the study (to prevent priming of memories prior to the memory task) using a standardised clinical interview (SCID) for the *Diagnostic and Statistical Manual for Mental Disorders* (*DSM-IV-TR*; American Psychiatric Association, 2001). One bipolar participant had to leave before the end of the study and was not available for the SCID. Participants were excluded if they fulfilled *DSM-IV-TR* criteria for a current episode of mania or depression. Participants who received a diagnosis of schizo-affective disorder were also excluded. The bipolar group reported significantly more episodes of depression than the unipolar group, but the two groups showed no significant differences in any of the remaining clinical and demographic variables summarised in Table 1. The standardised measures used were the Beck Depression Inventory (Beck, Ward, Mendelson, Mock, & Erbaugh,

TABLE 1
Characteristics of the sample

Clinical characteristic	Group		Statistic
	Bipolar (n = 19)	Unipolar (n = 16)	
Age	44.05 (13.88)	37.25 (10.76)	$t(33) = 1.60$
Female:male ratio	13:6	9:7	$\chi^2(1) = 0.43$
Years in education	16.00 (13.00 to 16.00)	16.00 (11.50 to 17.00)	$z = 0.26$
Beck Depression Inventory	7.00 (3.00 to 11.00)	8.00 (4.25 to 10.00)	$z = 0.43$
Hamilton Depression Scale	4.00 (3.00 to 7.00)	5.00 (3.00 to 5.75)	$z = 0.18$
Mania Rating Scale	1.00 (0 to 4.00)	5.00 (3.00 to 5.75)	$z = 1.61$
No. Episodes of Depression	6.00 (3.00 to 10.00)	1.00 (1.00 to 2.00)	$z = 4.75*$
			$r = 0.80$
No. Episodes of Mania	3.00 (2.00 to 10.00)	—	—
Past Comorbid Axis 1			$\chi^2(2) = 0.55$
None	9	8	
One	4	5	
Two or more	5	3	
Present Comorbid Axis 1			$\chi^2(2) = 2.07$
None	12	13	
One	4	3	
Two or more	2	0	

Standard deviations in brackets or interquartile range where the data are non-parametric.
$*p < .001$.

1961), the Hamilton Depression Scale (Hamilton, 1960), and the Mania Rating Scale (MRS; Bech, Rafaelson, Kramp, & Bolwig, 1978).

Procedure

Participants completed the standardised scales at home on the day of the study. They were told that they would be presented with two lists of four words. After being presented with each word list they were to tell the experimenter as soon as a memory of a specific event in their lives came to mind. The memory could be triggered by any of the four words on the list. One list contained positive words (optimistic, success, adored, confident) chosen from an earlier study to be relevant to bipolar affective disorder (Lam, Wright, & Sham, 2004a). The other list contained negative words that were antonyms to the positive words (pessimistic, failure, hated, unconfident). Participants were randomly allocated to view either the positive or the negative list first.

Following the identification of each memory, the experimenter asked the participant to rate the memory on several 7-point scales. They were adapted from an interview by Hackmann et al. (2000): how negative or positive is the memory? (-3 = "extremely negative" to $+3$ = "extremely

positive"); how exciting is the memory?; how anxious does it make you feel?; how distressing is this memory? (each rated from 0 = "not at all" to 6 = "extremely"). Next, the experimenter asked whether the memory involved an image that passed through their mind (Yes/No); otherwise, whether they had some other sensory impression of themselves or other people in the memory (Yes/No). If they had an image or impression, they next rated the memory on vividness (0 = "not at all" to 6 = "extremely"). The experimenter asked them to date the event relating to the memory and to estimate how often this memory normally came back to them in their everyday lives. Finally, the experimenter asked them to describe the memory, trying to recreate the scene or impression in as much detail as possible, describing what they saw, heard, or felt. Each memory was recorded on audiotape.

Each memory was coded as either specific, i.e., relating to a particular place and time, or general, i.e., a series of events over a period in the person's life or a kind of event (cf. Williams & Broadbent, 1986). A sample of 20 of the memories (10 positive and 10 negative) were coded independently by the experimenter and the second author (who was blind to experimental group). They met to discuss discrepant codings and these were recoded by discussion of the appropriate criteria. The experimenter then coded the remaining memories (as carried out by Willams & Broadbent, 1986), and the second author coded a sample of 20 of these to check for inter-rater reliability.

RESULTS

Overgeneral memory

The interrater reliability was sufficiently reliable ($j = 0.69$, $p < .001$, cf. Williams & Broadbent, 1986, $j = 0.68$, $p < .001$). The numbers of participants with each kind of memory were submitted to separate Group (bipolar – unipolar) × Category (general – specific) chi-squared tests for positive and negative memories. Following the prediction, the bipolar group reported significantly fewer specific negative memories ($f = 26\%$) than the unipolar group ($f = 75\%$), $\chi^2(1, N = 35) = 6.41$, $p < .05$, $w = 0.43$. See Table 2 for the exact numbers of each type of memory recalled. The effect for positive memories was in the predicted direction but it did not reach statistical significance, $\chi^2(1, N = 35) = 3.04$, $p = .081$, $w = 0.29$.

Imagery and specificity

All the memories recalled were submitted to an Image (yes–no) × Specificity (specific–general) chi-squared test to evaluate the prediction that specific memories would be more frequently associated with a mental image. The analysis of the association between images and specific memories revealed significant linear association for negative memories, $\chi^2(1, N = 35) = 4.44$, $p < .05$, $w = 0.75$, and positive memories, $\chi^2(1, N = 35) = 6.77$, $p < .01$, $w = 1.14$. Out of the 26 memories coded as general, 15 (56%) involved an image, whereas out of the 44 memories coded as specific, 41 (95%) involved an image.

Frequency of recollection in everyday life

The participants' responses to how frequently the memories usually came to mind in everyday life were converted to a standardised score of number of memories per month. Participants with memories less than a month old were excluded from the analysis. The scores were found to be significantly deviant from a normal distribution and so log transformations were computed. These figures were analysed using a Group (bipolar–unipolar) × Valence (positive–negative) ANOVA. This revealed a significant interaction, $F(1, 24) = 7.93$, $p < .05$, $MSE = 0.85$. Separate t-tests were carried out for the positive and negative memories. The bipolar group reported more frequent recollection of the negative past memory in everyday life than the unipolar group, $t(24) = 3.08$, $p < .01$, $d = 1.03$. This effect remained when repeating the analysis as a one-way ANOVA using number of past episodes of depression as a covariate, $F(1, 23) = 6.16$, $p < .05$, $MSE = 1.02$, $g^2 = 0.19$. There was no difference in the frequency of recollection of the positive memory in everyday life when comparing the bipolar group and the unipolar group, $t(25) = 0.82$, $p = .42$.

Properties

The properties of the negative and positive memories are displayed in Table 3. The participants' 7-point ratings of the properties of their recalled memory were found not to be normally distributed, and so log transformations were attempted, but the data remained significantly different from a normal distribution. Therefore, the ratings made by the participants were submitted to separate Group (bipolar–unipolar) Mann-Whitney U-tests for positive and negative memories. The participants' 7-point ratings of valence, excitement, anxiety, distress, and vividness were analysed, but no group differences were

TABLE 2

The number of negative and positive memories coded as specific versus general, and with or without an image, in each group of participants

Type of memory	Group	
	Bipolar	Unipolar
Negative memories		
General	14 (74%)	4 (25%)
With image	7	3
Without image	7	1
Specific	5 (26%)	12 (75%)
With image	3	12
Without image	2	0
Positive memories		
General	7 (37%)	1 (6%)
With image	4	1
Without image	3	0
Specific	12 (63%)	15 (94%)
With image	12	14
Without image	0	1

TABLE 3
The properties of the negative and positive memories in each experimental group

| | Group | | |
Property of the memory	Bipolar	Unipolar	Statistic
Negative memories			
Valence (−3 to +3)	−3.00 (−3.00 to −2.00)	−2.00 (−2.75 to −1.00)	$z = 1.62$
Exciting (0 to 6)	0.00 (0.00 to 0.00)	0.00 (0.00 to 0.00)	$z = 0.27$
Anxious (0 to 6)	3.00 (1.00 to 5.00)	2.00 (0 to 4.00)	$z = 1.33$
Distressing (0 to 6)	4.00 (1.00 to 5.00)	3.50 (0.25 to 4.00)	$z = 0.96$
Vivid (0 to 6)	5.00 (3.25 to 6.00)	5.00 (4.00 to 6.00)	$z = 0.37$
Recollections/month†	2.19 (0.20 to 5.50)	0.27 (0.02 to 1.00)	$t(24) = 3.08*$
Positive memories			
Valence (−3 to +3)	3.00 (2.00 to 3.00)	3.00 (2.25 to 3.00)	$z = 1.11$
Exciting (0 to 6)	5.00 (4.00 to 5.50)	5.00 (4.00 to 6.00)	$z = 0.77$
Anxious (0 to 6)	0.00 (0.00 to 0.00)	0.00 (0.00 to 0.75)	$z = 0.62$
Distressing (0 to 6)	0.00 (0.00 to 0.00)	0.00 (0.00 to 1.38)	$z = 0.92$
Vivid (0 to 6)	5.00 (3.00 to 6.00)	5.00 (4.00 to 6.00)	$z = 0.33$
Recollections/month†	0.21 (0.01 to 1.00)	0.40 (0.10 to 1.00)	$t(25) = 0.82$

Interquartile range in brackets.

$*p < .01$.

† Non-parametric data that were subject to parametric statistical tests after log transformation.

found (whether or not the alpha level was adjusted for multiple comparisons). Table 3 shows the medians, interquartile ranges, and statistics. The negative memories were rated by both groups of participants as vivid and moderately distressing. Characteristic examples of the memories that were recalled by the participants with remitted bipolar affective disorder are given in the Appendix.

DISCUSSION

We had predicted that the remitted bipolar group would recall more memories that were general rather than specific when compared to the remitted unipolar group. This prediction was confirmed for negative memories with a near-significant trend for positive memories. This result tentatively extends the findings of Scott et al. (2000) to suggest that patients with remitted bipolar disorder have a higher frequency of general memories than remitted unipolar patients as well as compared to healthy controls. In our sample, the bipolar patients had significantly more past depressive episodes than the unipolar patients. This suggests that overgeneral memory is not a result of having experienced depression *per se*, but may be related to having a psychological disorder

that is prone to relapses of mania and depression, namely bipolar disorder.

This study also investigated the role of imagery in recalling specific memories. Across both groups, specific memories were much more likely to be associated with images than general memories. This finding supports the notion that the retrieval of specific events may often be accompanied by imagery. Interestingly, around half of the general memories also involved a mental image. Thus, a mental image is not a sufficient criterion for a memory to be specific. In some cases, the mental image may represent a convergence of a whole period or theme within an individual's life (as in the descriptions of the experiences of depression in the Appendix). As explained earlier, in their model of autobiographical memory, Conway and Pleydell-Pearce (2000) explain that repeated incidences of traumatic events can form an accumulated structure of "event-specific knowledge" (ESK) that is triggered by related goals. ESK is sensory-perceptual in nature and therefore may correspond to the crystallised images of repeated events reported by the patients in this study.

The remitted bipolar group reported that the negative memories they had identified were recollected more often in everyday life, compared to the unipolar group. This finding remained even when taking account of the greater number of past episodes of depression in the bipolar group. This finding adds remitted bipolar disorder to the list of psychological disorders that are associated with an elevated frequency of vivid distressing memories. Notably, positive memories showed no significant effect in that there was no group difference in their frequency of recollection in everyday life. We had predicted that the remitted bipolar group would report a higher frequency of recollections of the positive memory. The absence of this effect suggests the possibility that the high mood experienced in bipolar disorder may not associated with positive memories. Indeed, there may be theoretical reasons, described in more detail later, that high mood may be more closely associated with negative memories.

The contents of the memories were not reported in detail, but it appears that several bipolar participants reported memories relating to failures at personal goals and to the experience of depression (see Appendix). Failure in highly valued goals may be particularly likely to lead to depression in bipolar disorder. This hypothesis is yet to be explored in any detail. Taken together, the results suggest that remitted bipolar patients experience the kinds of biases in autobiographical memory that are also associated with current unipolar depression. This indicates that they may benefit from cognitive therapy interventions that are known to be effective in unipolar depression. Many treatment protocols already include components aimed at tackling cognitive biases associated with depression (e.g., Lam, Jones, Hayward, & Bright, 1999; Lam et al., 2004a).

One possible explanation for the finding that remitted bipolar patients show similar cognitive biases to people with unipolar depression may be that they are in fact currently depressed, and the fact that they do not explicitly present as depressed is a form of denial or "manic-defence" (e.g. Dooley, 1921). For example, Winters and Neale (1985) found that people with remitted bipolar disorder show high levels of social desirability, an index of defensiveness. We think that the "manic-defence" explanation does not necessarily follow from our findings. First, the participants in this study were not currently experiencing mania and so the proposal that mania itself may act as a defence could not be tested directly. Second, the patients were not completely in denial of depression, in that they did explicitly admit to low levels of depressive symptoms.

Even though the manic-defence account may not directly explain the findings, it is possible that the processing of negative recurrent memories may have some role in the escalation or maintenance of manic symptoms. Returning to theories of autobiographical memory, Conway and Pleydell-Pearce (2000) propose that ESK is associated with the working goals of the self. Therefore, the active pursuit of goals triggers the retrieval of these memories. For example, a person with PTSD may have narrowly escaped severe injury when an approaching lorry careered into the side of her car. Long after the accident, she may still experience distressing ESKs of the approaching lorry when she engages in the goal of trying to drive for the first time. Applying this model to bipolar disorder, one might predict that negative intrusive memories around themes of past personal failure would be more likely to be triggered when people with bipolar disorder strive to achieve personal goals of success and high social status. Recent studies of the role of early memories in psychological disorder (e.g., social phobia; Hackmann et al., 2000), suggest that the nature of the processing of these kinds of memories would be critical; if patients appraise memories of failure as a reflection of the *current* situation, then they may think that they need to continue in the present to try as hard as possible in order to prevent being seen as a failure by other people. However, they would be responding to memories rather than the current situation. Therefore, their behaviour may escalate and seem inappropriate to the social context.

Conway and Pleydell-Pearce (2000) argue that the way to prevent distressing ESK from being triggered is to integrate it with the remaining autobiographical knowledge base. Indeed, this account is consistent with models and clinical interventions within PTSD (Brewin & Holmes, 2003; Ehlers & Clark, 2000; Grey, Young, & Holmes, 2002). Thus, it may be the case that a suitable treatment for bipolar disorder would be to elicit the negative memories that are triggered during goal-directed behaviour and promote their cognitive restructuring and integration. It is notable that the cognitive restructuring of distressing memories typically requires patients to relive the experience, or to hold an image of the specific event in mind. Thus, an important step in therapy is the access of *specific* memories rather than general memories (whereas general memories were identified at high rates within the remitted bipolar group in this study). Therapy then often involves introducing contextual information into the memory that allows the memory to be integrated with other autobiographical knowledge. For example, a patient with bipolar disorder always felt that she was not good enough when trying to perform at work, leading her to work extremely hard and relapse. Through Socratic questioning it was discovered that this belief related to the repeated experience throughout her childhood of her father criticising but never praising her when he taught her mathematics at home. She experienced ESKs of this situation when involved in her work. The therapist asked the patient to hold her ESK of this experience in mind, and asked the patient to choose contextual information to bring into the memory. It included the fact that the patient's father had in fact told her during adulthood that he had actually been pleased with her when she was a child, and that she now realised that her father thought he was doing the best for her by not praising her. Naturally, these clinical suggestions and their theoretical foundations are preliminary at this stage and require further investigation.

This study is preliminary and has several limitations. The sample size was small and entailed many non-parametric statistics. Therefore future studies could use a larger sample. The memory task used had many different components and therefore it was not identical to any one study in the pre-existing literature. This held an advantage in that autobiographical memory could be explored from many perspectives, but held the disadvantage that the study may not be measuring exactly the same constructs as earlier research. The adapted memory interview used was not independently evaluated for reliability and validity, and was different from the original version in that the ratings were carried out before, rather than after, the description of the memory. The coding of the memories was not carried out blind to experimental group, but it was verified by a rater who was blind to patient's group status. This method has clear precedent in the literature (e.g., Williams & Broadbent, 1986), but it is not ideal. The bipolar group in this study had had many more episodes of depression than the unipolar group in this study. We demonstrated that this difference could not account for the increased frequency of recollections of negative past memories in the remitted bipolar group. Nevertheless, future studies could try to match bipolar and unipolar groups on the number of past episodes of depression. They could also include a never-depressed healthy control group in order to further identify processes in bipolar affective disorder that are either unique to the disorder, or shared with unipolar depression but not present in people who have never been depressed. Despite the limitations of this study, it provides some indication that bipolar affective disorder is a fruitful area of research into autobiographical memory.

REFERENCES

American Psychiatric Association. (2001). *The Diagnostic and Statistical Manual for Mental Disorders* (4th ed., text revision). Washington, DC: American Psychiatric Association.

Bebbington, P., & Ramana, R. (1995). The epidemiology of bipolar affective disorder. *Social Psychiatry and Psychiatric Epidemiology*, *30*, 279–292.

Bech, P., Rafaelson, O. J., Kramp, P., & Bolwig, T. G. (1978). The Mania Rating Scale: Scale construction and inter-observer agreement. *Neuropharmacology*, *17*, 430–431.

Beck, A. T., Ward, C., Mendelson, M., Mock, J., & Erbaugh, J. (1961). An inventory for measuring depression. *Archives of General Psychiatry*, *4*, 561–567.

Brewin, C. R., & Holmes, E. A. (2003). Psychological theories of posttraumatic stress disorder. *Clinical Psychology Review*, *23*, 339–376.

Brittlebank, A. D., Scott, J., Williams, J. M. G., & Ferrier, I. N. (1993). Autobiographical memory in depression: State or trait marker? *British Journal of Psychiatry*, *162*, 118–121.

Conway, M. A., & Pleydell-Pearce, C. W. (2000). The construction of autobiographical memory in the self-memory system. *Psychological Review*, *107*, 261–288.

Conway, M. A., Pleydell-Pearce, C. W., & Whitecross, S. (2001). The neuroanatomy of autobiographical memory: A slow cortical potential study (SCP) of autobiographical memory retrieval. *Journal of Memory and Language*, *45*, 493–524.

Dooley, L. (1921). A psychoanalytic study of manic-depressive psychosis. *Psychoanalytic Review*, *8*, 38–72.

Ehlers, A., & Clark, D. M. (2000). A cognitive model of posttraumatic stress disorder. *Behaviour Research and Therapy*, *38*, 319–345.

Ehlers, A., Hackmann, A., Steil, R., Clohessy, S., Wenninger, K., & Winter, H. (2002). The nature of intrusive memories after trauma: The warning signal hypothesis. *Behaviour Research and Therapy*, *40*, 995–1002.

Evans, J., Williams, J. M. G., O'Loughlin, S., & Howells, K. (1992). Autobiographical memory and problem solving strategies of individuals who parasuicide. *Psychological Medicine*, *22*, 399–405.

Goodwin, F. K., & Jamison, K. R. (1990). *Manic-depressive illness*. New York: Oxford University Press.

Grey, N., Young, K., & Holmes, E. A. (2002). Cognitive restructuring within reliving: A treatment for peritraumatic emotional "hotspots" in posttraumatic stress disorder. *Behavioural and Cognitive Psychotherapy*, *30*, 37–56.

Hackmann, A., Clark, D. M., & McManus, F. (2000). Recurrent images and early memories in social phobia. *Behaviour Research & Therapy*, *38*, 601–610.

Hamilton, M. (1960). A rating scale for depression. *Journal of Neurology and Psychiatry*, *23*, 56–62.

Lam, D. H., Jones, S. H., Hayward, P., & Bright, J. A. (1999). *Cognitive therapy for bipolar disorder: A therapist's guide to concepts, methods and practice.* Chichester, UK: Wiley.

Lam, D. H., Watkins, E. R., Hayward, P., Bright, J., Wright, K., Kerr, N. et al. (2003). A randomised controlled trial of cognitive therapy of relapse prevention for bipolar affective disorder: Outcome of the first year. *Archives of General Psychiatry*, *60*, 145–152.

Lam, D. H., Wright, K., & Sham, P. (2004a). *Sense of hyper-positive self and response to cognitive therapy for bipolar affective disorder.* Manuscript submitted for publication.

Lam, D. H., Wright, K., & Smith, N. (2004b). Dysfunctional attitudes: Extreme goal-attainment beliefs in remitted bipolar patients. *Journal of Affective Disorders*, *79*, 193–199.

McNally, R. J., Lasko, N. B., Macklin, M. L., & Pitman, R. K. (1995). Autobiographical memory disturbance in combat-related post-traumatic stress disorder. *Behaviour Research and Therapy*, *33*, 619–630.

Morrison, A. P., Beck, A. T., Glentworth, D., Dunn, H., Reid, G. S., Larkin, W. et al. (2002). Imagery and psychotic symptoms: A preliminary investigation. *Behaviour Research and Therapy*, *40*, 1053–1062.

Norman, D. A., & Brobrow, D. G. (1979). Descriptions: An intermediate stage in memory retrieval. *Cognitive Psychology*, *11*, 107–123.

Reynolds, M., & Brewin, C. R. (1999). Intrusive memories in depression and posttraumatic stress disorder. *Behaviour Research and Therapy*, *37*, 201–215.

Robins, L. N., Helzer, J. E., Weissman, M. M., Orvaschel , H., Gruenberg, E., Burke, J. D. et al. (1984). Lifetime prevalence of specific psychiatric disorders in three sites. *Archives of General Psychiatry*, *41*, 949–958.

Scott, J., Stanton, B., Garland, A., & Ferrier, I. N. (2000). Cognitive vulnerability in patients with bipolar disorder. *Psychological Medicine*, *30*, 467–472.

Tohen, M., Waternaux, C. M., & Tsuang, M. T. (1990). Outcome in mania: A 4-year prospective follow-up of 75 patients utilizing survival analysis. *Archives of General Psychiatry*, *47*, 1106–1111.

Wells, A., & Hackmann, A. (1993). Imagery and core beliefs in health anxiety: Contents and origins. *Behavioural & Cognitive Psychotherapy*, *21*, 265–273.

Williams, J. M. G. (1996). Memory processes in psychotherapy. In P. M. Salkovskis (Ed.), *Frontiers of cognitive therapy* (pp. 97–113). New York: Guilford Press.

Williams, J. M. G., & Broadbent, K. (1986). Autobiographical memory in suicide attempters. *Journal of Abnormal Psychology*, *95*, 144–149.

Williams, J. M. G., & Dritschel, B. H. (1988). Emotional disturbance and the specificity of autobiographical memory. *Cognition and Emotion*, *2*, 221–234.

Williams, J. M. G., Healy, H. G., & Ellis, N. C. (1999). The effect of imageability and predicability of cues in autobiographical memory. *Quarterly Journal of Experimental Psychology*, *52*A, 555–579.

Williams, J. M. G., & Scott, J. (1988). Autobiographical memory in depression. *Psychological Medicine*, *18*, 689–695.

Winters, K. C., & Neale, J. M. (1985). Mania and low self-esteem. *Journal of Abnormal Psychology*, *94*, 282–290.

APPENDIX

Examples of autobiographical memories recalled by participants with remitted bipolar affective disorder (imagery descriptions are reproduced in italics)

Several memories related to failing at the pursuit of important personal goals:

"I went to [college to do] something completely different so it was a big challenge and I set myself up to work very, very, very hard for the whole year, but that was the only way I was going to get through and I did work very hard ... so I felt that I was capable at what I was doing but I was handicapped by lack of background, but also a lot of things to do with the environment that I was put in by other people rather than myself and the environment that existed already there and that I came off on the bad side of a lot of those things, so I felt that I succeeded in a lot of ways but in terms of actual recognition or results to go home with it wasn't, it didn't work out at all, and there were a lot of negative things I came away with in terms of the place and some of the people in it as well ..."

"The word which prompted the memory was failure, and it was actually my French master at school relating to me something which the History master had said about me in the staff room. I was very good at History. I got a scholarship. I had to sit with him all that year, just the two of us but we never had the eye contact and he accepted from this that I was going to be a failure in life, in life generally. I was told he said that but I'm not sure why the French master told me that. It pissed me off, you know, but, and when I'm depressed I think of this, so it does come back quite often. *I have a very big image of sitting there for over three quarters of an hour and not being able to get eye contact, trying but not getting any, and he had a bald head, and constantly looking round his head to see what time it was. He did not want to be there with me.*"

"My mother being her usual self when I've done something or achieved something or whatever and it didn't have any value, and she was constantly referring to me as a failure and not as good as my siblings and stuff like that."

Five memories in the remitted bipolar group (but none in the unipolar group) related to past experiences of depression and included:

"This memory ... reminds me of a time 18 months ago when I was clinically depressed, and at a point where I didn't sort of want to exist, where even breathing was painful because it meant that I existed and I can remember just when seconds just seemed to last for hours and lying on the bed in the middle of the night, being just very awake and just existing and existing being the most painful thing I'd experienced ... *The image would be, would just be me looking at a clock, experiencing time and thinking it would never end.*"

"*The image I have flashes of memory of is of me being in bed during the day with no sense of relevance to the world*, so it's not a positive, it's not really a strong negative feeling. It's not really strong depression. It's a sense of antipathy and placelessness, having no purpose, because ordinarily what I do I believe strongly in, in the stuff that I work on, and it's what I research as well, so my usual feeling is that I have a role to play ... where I would be happy would be if I'd just fallen asleep and just woken up and realised that about an hour had passed by and I hadn't had to engage with anything. I hadn't had to think, and its just wishing time away really."

Images of desire: Cognitive models of craving

Jon May, Jackie Andrade, and Nathalie Panabokke

University of Sheffield, UK

David Kavanagh

University of Queensland, Australia

Cognitive modelling of phenomena in clinical practice allows the operationalisation of otherwise diffuse descriptive terms such as craving or flashbacks. This supports the empirical investigation of the clinical phenomena and the development of targeted treatment interventions. This paper focuses on the cognitive processes underpinning craving, which is recognised as a motivating experience in substance dependence. We use a high-level cognitive architecture, Interacting Cognitive Subsystems (ICS), to compare two theories of craving: Tiffany's theory, centred on the control of automated action schemata, and our own Elaborated Intrusion theory of craving. Data from a questionnaire study of the subjective aspects of everyday desires experienced by a large non-clinical population are presented. Both the data and the high-level modelling support the central claim of the Elaborated Intrusion theory that imagery is a key element of craving, providing the subjective experience and mediating much of the associated disruption of con-current cognition.

When I get to work in the morning, I almost always have an intense urge to have a cup of coffee. Sometimes it comes to me almost like I am talking to myself—"I must get a cup of coffee before I do anything else". Sometimes I look at my coffee cup and imagine it is filled with coffee. Sometimes my mouth feels dry, and I can imagine what it will be like to have a drink. I get these thoughts and feelings whether or not I have already had a cup at home, and I find it hard to concentrate on anything else without getting that cup of coffee first.

ADVANTAGES OF A COGNITIVE APPROACH TO CLINICAL DISORDERS

Craving is popularly recognised as a powerful subjective experience that motivates people to seek out and use or consume a craved substance. It has long been identified as an important symptom in addictive disorders (Jellinek, 1960), but the subjective experience of craving is not well explained by current conditioning and neuro-chemical theories. These see craving as a consequence of learned physiological responses to cues in the world or the body, perhaps predisposed by individual differences in neurochemistry, leading to the activation of schematised action plans. By focusing on the antecedent states of the body and the neurophysiological consequences of those states, these models do not address what is happening, mentally, during a craving episode. The subjective aspects are seen as secondary, because consumption and craving are both caused by the same physical events: the feelings that are experienced during a craving episode do not cause people to consume, but are a by-product of the addictive process. On the other hand, the need for a cognitive account of craving that does address the subjective aspects of craving is illustrated by evidence that pharmacological treatments for substance abuse work through their effects on

Correspondence should be sent to Jon May, Department of Psychology, University of Sheffield, Sheffield UK. Email: jon.may@shef.ac.uk craving (Monti et al., 1999; O'Malley, Krishnan-Sarin, Farren, Sinha, & Kreek, 2002) and do so most effectively when combined with cognitive behavioural therapy (Monti et al., 2001; O'Malley et al., 1996). Understanding the cognitive processes underlying craving may help to improve treatments for substance dependence, by allowing us to influence the mental and subjective aspects of those cravings that occur despite pharmacological intervention. In turn, understanding craving in substance dependence may help to improve our understanding of normal, non-addictive states of desire. In this paper we outline two cognitive accounts of craving, and use an information processing framework called Interacting Cognitive Subsystems (ICS; Barnard, 1985; May, 2001) to model and compare them. We then evaluate the models against data from a questionnaire in which a large sample were asked to describe the subjective nature of an everyday craving.

In general, cognitive theories allow the operationalisation of otherwise diffuse, descriptive terms. By incorporating clinical phenomena into established theories of cognition, this operationalisation supports the empirical investigation of the clinical phenomena, and the development of targeted treatment interventions. Building a cognitive model of a phenomenon requires the theorist to specify what processes are and are not involved, and inspection of the model allows inferences to be drawn concerning processing consequences that follow logically from the model. In this way the model can contribute to the scientific process by making clear whether a theory is self-consistent (i.e., whether it can in fact be modelled), and by identifying empirical tests that might not have been apparent from the theory itself.

We have previously used a cognitive approach to examine Eye Movement Desensitisation-Reprocessing (EMD-R), which has gained some popularity as a treatment for post-traumatic stress disorder (PTSD). In PTSD, vivid, lifelike images of trauma (called flashbacks) are a diagnostic symptom. EMD-R involves the use of eye movements during a type of imaginal desensitisation. While eye movements have not been found to amplify average treatment effects, we predicted from cognitive theory and research that they may have some utility. Using Baddeley and Hitch's (1974; Baddeley, 1986) model of working memory as a theoretical framework, we hypothesised that tasks loading on either the phonological loop or the visuospatial sketchpad would reduce the

vividness of mental imagery in the same modality. We demonstrated that this was the case (Baddeley & Andrade, 2000), and also that there was a concomitant reduction in the reported emotional response to the images and memories (Andrade, Kavanagh, & Baddeley, 1997; Kavanagh, Freese, Andrade, & May, 2001). We have suggested (Kavanagh et al., 2001) that carefully chosen working memory loads may be a useful treatment aid when designing stepwise exposure protocols for the treatment of post-traumatic stress disorder.

The EMD-R studies illustrate the potential that cognitive psychology has to explain the mode of action of clinical treatments, and to refine them to increase their effectiveness. They also illustrate that the development of cognitive explanations of clinical phenomena can be beneficial to cognitive psychology. The finding of reductions in image vividness and emotionality raised theoretical questions about the link between the working memory processes thought to underlie imagery, and emotion. The subjective nature of craving is another topic offering a potentially fruitful overlap between clinical and cognitive approaches. As in the case of traumatic imagery, it raises questions about the relationship between cognition and emotion, and specifically the role that mental imagery plays in craving.

A COGNITIVE APPROACH TO CRAVING

Craving appears to be a major cause of the discomfort experienced by people trying to reduce their substance use, and subjectively is a factor in triggering relapse. While its actual causal role in relapse is disputed, the evidence suggests it is indeed one of several determinants. For example Killen and Fortmann (1997) found highly significant relationships between the craving of 2600 former smokers and their relapse over the subsequent 12 months.

We have proposed the Elaborated Intrusion (EI) theory of craving, (Kavanagh, Andrade, & May, 2004) which aims to explain the cognitive processes underlying craving episodes, and to explain the emotional and motivational impact of these processes. In particular, we argue that craving episodes persist because cravers create mental images of the desired substance that are immediately pleasurable but which exacerbate their awareness of deficit. This causes a vicious circle of desire, imagery, and planning to satisfy that desire, followed by greater articulation of the imagery that engages high-level cognitive processes (e.g., working memory), impairs performance on concurrent cognitive tasks, and amplifies the emotional response. Our approach assumes that craving for addictive substances such as nicotine and alcohol is an extreme instance of a range of normal phenomena associated with motivated consumption behaviours.

A craving episode is shown in Figure 1. Any of several triggers can give rise to cognitive activity below the threshold of awareness, which can then trigger other associations. These do not have any specific consequences until they break through

into awareness, when they are experienced as intrusive thoughts. These feel spontaneous because the triggers and the prior processing have been acting beneath awareness. Because the thoughts contain information that is linked to the use of some substance, there is an initial immediate positive sensation of reward or relief, as there would be if the substance were actually being used (a conditioned positive affective response). This encourages the individual to elaborate the thought, to enrich it, and to search for further associations, which are in turn also rewarding. We argue that the elaboration process particularly involves the construction of mental

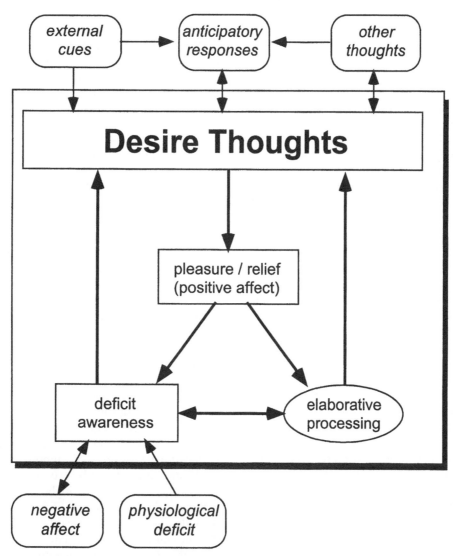

Figure 1.   The Elaborated Intrusion theory (Kavanagh et al.). Antecedents of a craving episode are shown in rounded boxes outside the central box, which represents a craving episode. Cognitive products are indicated by rectangles and processing by an ellipse. Elaborative Processing includes the construction and elaboration of images of the target and its consumption. The consequences of craving (i.e., consumption or avoidance actions) are not shown in this figure.

images of the substance or of its context of consumption, and it is these images that provide the strongest reward and relief. Semantic and verbal elaborations are also involved, but do not necessarily have the same affective consequences.

This process of elaboration following intrusion is the key to our theory, and in normal situations it motivates an individual to seek out some substance that they may need to obtain. In maladaptive situations, it can lead them to seek out substances that they do not need, or are even attempting to avoid consuming. In these cases the elaborated thoughts soon lead to negative affective consequences as the individual realises the conflict with their goal of abstention, and they may attempt to control the elaboration by thought suppression or diversion (with limited success, or even increased elaboration, as in Wegner's ironic processes, 1994). In other cases, the individual may not want to control their consumption, but may be prevented from obtaining the substance by circumstances or by its non-availability. In this case the rewarding consequences of the elaborated thoughts are soon overcome by the negative realisation of their growing deficit state, which is made increasingly salient by the content of their thoughts.

Memory plays a key role in the EI theory of craving, because the processes of elaboration are essentially a goal-driven search through long-term memory for associations of the intrusive thoughts. The mediating mental representations that give rise to the subjective phenomenological aspects of craving are argued to be mental images arising from this elaborative search. The theory was informed by earlier research showing the role of working memory (WM) in imagery (e.g., Baddeley & Andrade, 2000), but the WM model does not explain the link between imagery and emotion demonstrated by Andrade et al. (1997) and Kavanagh et al. (2001) and assumed in the EI theory of craving. This is simply because Baddeley and Hitch's (1974) WM model was only constructed as a model of short-term memory and its use in complex cognition, and there is no scope within the model for accounts of other phenomena. Emotional consequences of activity with the WM model are unspecified, and so this model does not provide any support for reasoning about the subjective nature of craving.

An information processing approach to cognition that does include an explicit account of the relationship between cognition and emotion is Barnard's (1985) Interacting Cognitive Sub-

systems (ICS). Because of this it has been applied to a range of clinical phenomena, and provides a high-level framework for explaining the cognitive processes involved in such conditions. Whereas the EI theory is only concerned with craving, ICS provides a way of modelling how craving might interact with other clinical problems. This modelling may help to design treatment interventions for complex problems such as comorbidities of substance abuse and psychological disorders such as schizophrenia or depression. As a general-purpose architecture for cognition, it can also help theorists to relate different accounts of a single phenomenon that have been motivated by different considerations, but which may overlap. Here we attempt an initial interpretation of the EI theory within the ICS architecture, to compare it with an influential cognitive theory of craving (Tiffany, 1990), which incorporates the cognitive interference phenomenon but de-emphasises emotional aspects and argues that craving is epiphenomenal to substance use.

AN INTERACTING COGNITIVE SUBSYSTEMS APPROACH

We need first to briefly introduce the essential points of the ICS architecture (more detailed accounts are available in Teasdale & Barnard, 1993, and May, 2001), highlighting key theoretical terms in italics. ICS is a representational theory of mind, in which thought is divided into nine different types of representation, each with a specific quality of informational content (see Figure 2 for descriptions). Cognitive processes transform information from one type of representation into another, qualitatively changing it through interactions with memory. Cognition is a configuration of activity distributed across the overall architecture. The nine subsystems operate upon sensory (visual, acoustic, and body state), effector (articulatory and limb), perceptual (object and morphonolexical), and central (propositional and implicational) levels of representation. The implicational level will be crucial for our models of craving: it consists of high-level, connotative schemata that contain the abstract meaning for the individual of particular situations or events. Its flavour can best be appreciated by contrasting it with the factual and semantic nature of the propositional level. Making a qualitative judgement about something requires the implicational level; making a quantitative or comparative

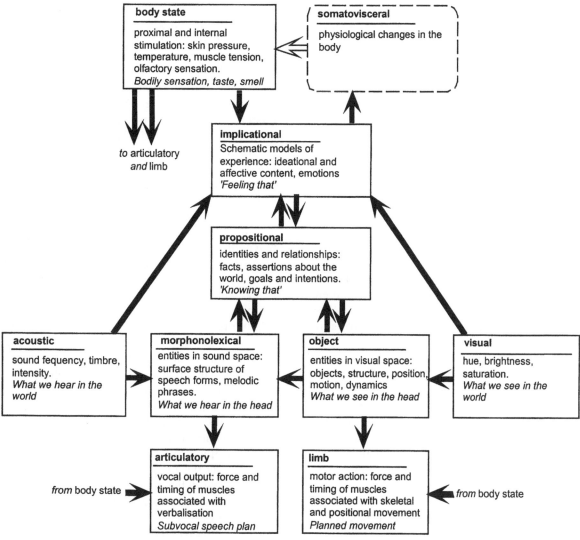

Figure 2. The nine levels of representation in ICS are shown in the rectangular boxes, each box corresponding to a single subsystem. The arrows indicate processes by which one representation can be transformed into another. The somatovisceral changes caused by the implicational subsystem are physiological rather than cognitive, and so there is no somatovisceral subsystem to process or memorise them; however, they can be detected by the body state subsystem, as indicated by the white arrow.

judgement requires the propositional level. The distinction between "hot" implicational and "cold" propositional representations is perhaps the hallmark of ICS.

Despite the different classes of information represented at each level in ICS, the nine subsystems carry out the same generic information processing activities, and share a common architecture. Each consists of an *input array*, which receives representations produced for it by other subsystems (or the senses); a *copy process*, which writes the contents of the input array into the subsystem's *image record*, which thus acts as a memory for everything the subsystem has ever received; and a set of *transformation processes*, which operate upon either the contents of the input array or the contents of the image record that have been activated as a result of the copy process (i.e., revived memories). Each subsystem contains two or three transformation processes (indicated by the arrows in Figure 2), meaning that not all subsystems can exchange representations directly.

Memories and processing develop over time so that the transformation processes accrue sets of *proceduralised knowledge* that allow them to produce an output representation directly from patterns on the input array without accessing memories in the image record. Before this has occurred, however, they do need to access the image record, and only one of the transformations within a subsystem can access its image record at a time. There is thus competition with subsystems for memory access. When the information being processed is particularly uncertain or hard for a transformation to operate upon, a subsystem can enter buffered processing mode, whereby the information being copied into the image record is re-accessed by the transformation a few moments later, providing an integration of the information over the very short term. ICS theory allows only one buffer to be active at any moment, and so there is competition between subsystems for buffered processing mode. While the copy process within each subsystem gives rise to a sense of diffuse awareness for the information it is processing, buffered processing gives rise to a focal sense of awareness of the information. Because there is only one buffer active at any moment, focal awareness has a unitary nature, although its quality can vary depending on the level of representation being buffered.

Memory is a key resource in ICS, in terms of the individual components of the architecture (the image records of the subsystems, and procedural knowledge within the transformation processes, for example), and the dynamics of their interaction (the limited access to the image record within each subsystem, and especially the single focus of buffered processing within a configuration).

AN ICS MODEL OF THE EI THEORY

An ICS model of the EI theory is a process-based account which specifies the memory resources that are required to be active from moment to moment in an episode of craving. The architecture within which any model is built contributes its own constraints and organisation to a less well specified theoretical account of a phenomenon. This specification helps us to be more precise and hence allows us to make detailed predictions about the interaction of craving with other cognitive activities, and in particular, to predict how other activities may interfere with craving. These predictions could perhaps have been made without an ICS, or any other, model of the theory, and once they have been made, they may seem obvious. Nevertheless, the fact that the process-based account did help in their derivation is in itself justification for the modelling process, and it also provides a rationale for the predictions. If the predictions are not supported by subsequent

empirical investigation, the rationale can be inspected, and possible explanations examined step by step, to repair either the model (if it was an inaccurate representation of the theory) or the theory (if the model was accurate). Without a model, failure to support a theoretical prediction leaves us none the wiser about how to improve a theory. The triggers postulated as eliciting a craving episode in the EI theory of craving could in principle arise at any of the nine levels of representation in ICS. External cues would be sensed and then represented at the visual or acoustic levels. Highly proceduralised knowledge in the visual–object and acoustic–morphonolexical transformation processes would lead to perceptual representations being formed (at an object and a morphonolexical level respectively); these could then lead to propositional information being generated via object–propositional or morphonolexical–propositional transformations.

Alternatively, the visual–implicational and acoustic–implicational processes might generate information in the high-level schematic representation. This might lead to the implicational–somatovisceral process driving changes in the individual's physiological state, which could be detected as body state representations and, via the body state–implicational transformation, lead to a change in mood. Similar chains of activity could be triggered by the body state subsystem detecting physiological deficits, or could be triggered in a purely cognitive manner, by processes that are not currently in use as part of the configuration supporting the individual's primary task.

Processes that are involved in a primary task configuration, but which are momentarily inactive, can be caught up in secondary configurations. Depending on the richness of the representations available for processing, and the degree of proceduralisation, cognitive activity can oscillate between primary and secondary tasks. If the secondary configuration is coherent enough, then a lacuna in the primary configuration can allow it to enter buffered processing and break through into focal awareness, in effect becoming the primary configuration. Subjectively, the individual will have had an intrusion into awareness of a thought not necessarily related to their previous chain of thought. This is the first specific contribution that ICS makes to the EI model: the definition of the conditions under which nonconscious cognitive processing can become conscious. This is the moment at which a person becomes aware of a craving, in the EI theory.

The next stage in a craving episode is for the intrusive thought to lead to reward or relief due to its similarity to the real substance. This is where the ICS model makes its second specific contribution, by a limitation on the pathways that can give rise to reward and relief. In ICS these affective states come about through the elicitation of an implicational schema concerned with the substance, and the consequent somatovisceral changes. Intrusive representations will be most likely to result in reward and relief if they directly allow the formation of implicational representations, and only the three sensory subsystems and the propositional subsystem can do this. The object and morphonolexical subsystems cannot produce implicational representations directly, and so intrusions there would need to involve a two-step sequence by first creating a propositional representation, followed by a propositional–implicational transformation. Intrusions in the two effector subsystems would only reach awareness if they conflicted with ongoing behavioural output, resulting in an action slip (Norman, 1981) at the limb level or a Freudian slip at the articulatory level.

A third, and perhaps the most testable, contribution of the ICS model comes from the consequences of the activation of the implicational schema for a substance. If this substance is one that the individual has habitually used, then the existence of procedural knowledge would lead to the elaboration of propositional representations for obtaining and using the substance, followed by the generation of morphonolexical or object level targets controlling these behaviours. These correspond to the generation of verbal and visual images of the substance, respectively. Both are feasible, and which predominated would depend on the nature of the tasks involved in searching for and using the substance. In consequence, it can be predicted that where the task involved physical movement and acquisition of a discrete spatially locatable substance, a triad of implicational, propositional, and object representations would dominate thought, with focal awareness oscillating between mental visual images of the substance and the affective implications of its use. This functionally based emphasis on object-level visual imagery is consistent with the EI model, but is not a necessary part of it, and so is a prediction drawn from the model of the theory (and hence from ICS) rather than from the theory itself.

Summarising this, the ICS account sees secondary configurations of cognitive activity arising as a result of unattended activity in the cognitive system. Processes that are not involved in the current primary task can generate a stream of processing that can break into awareness if the proceduralisation of associated processing is strong enough and the primary task is not demanding enough to retain processing resources. Crucial for the intrusion to gain control is the elicitation of an implicational level of representation concerning the craved substance, which will lead to both a somatovisceral response (if this has not already been part of the precursor activity) and mental imagery, which further supports the maintenance of the implicational representation. This activity places heavy demands on the two central subsystems, effectively taking control of thought and precluding other cognitive activity.

TIFFANY'S THEORY IN ICS TERMS

Tiffany's (1990) account of craving is also based on a general distinction between automatic and non-automatic cognitive processing, although he steps back from any particular theoretical definition of automaticity. In general, he points out that non-automatic processes are seen as those that require cognitive effort and control for execution, are strategic, and involve conscious awareness of choices and execution. They are constrained by competition for cognitive resources, and so only a single sequence of non-automatic processing can be carried out at a single moment. In contrast, automatic processes develop through practice, can be carried out without cognitive effort, and are not resource limited. Importantly for Tiffany, they can be executed without requiring conscious control, and are in fact difficult to control, having an aspect of cognitive impenetrability. Repeated drug use leads to the development of action schemata: overlearned, automatic patterns of behaviour directed towards the acquisition and consumption of a particular substance. These schemata are elicited by certain patterns of external and internal sensory stimuli, and contain coordinated sequences of actions, organised with alternative sequences to overcome common obstacles. Included within the schemata are physiological responses that support the motor behaviour required, and the generation of physiological adjustments in anticipation of drug consumption. In practice, the schemata allow the user to obtain and consume their substance with minimum cognitive effort, without distracting them from other cognitive activity, and prepare them for the physiological demands and effects of drug use.

Tiffany's action schemata for drug use do not inevitably lead to craving. Craving is a consequence of their failure to operate. This can be either because some situation arises in the course of their execution which is not covered by the learned set of alternative action sequences, or because the user is attempting to abstain from drug use, and so inhibiting their execution. Although the subsequent goals and behaviours differ, in both cases non-automatic cognitive processing becomes involved, and the user becomes aware of the situation. They will find that awareness of the physiological responses cued by the action schemata interferes with their non-automatic, controlled behaviour, giving a subjective characteristic to craving episodes that is not present when other, non-drug related action schemata are blocked or inhibited.

In ICS, the development of action schemata is well specified. Automatic processes correspond to those for which a high level of proceduralised knowledge is available within transformation processes. Given an appropriate input representation, a transformation process can operate immediately and directly to produce an output representation, without needing to access its image record. When sequential transformation processes in different subsystems have been repeatedly engaged in a particular task, the whole sequence can become proceduralised. This has several consequences. First, the absence of image record access means that the schemata can be carried out simultaneously with other configurations of cognitive activity that use different transformations. Second, there is no need for any of the subsystems to enter into buffered processing, and so if other less well proceduralised processing is ongoing, the action schemata will not enter focal awareness. Third, over the course of proceduralisation, loops of cognitive processing will be replaced by direct processing, so that gradually the involvement of the central subsystems will become minimised. For example, a simple visuo-motor task might initially involve a sequence of visual to object, and object to limb transformations, with a loop between the object to propositional levels serving to clarify the identity of the object representation. With practice, the procedural knowledge in the object–limb transformation would develop to the point that it becomes able to operate directly on the representation provided by the visual–object process,

and the need for involvement of the propositional subsystem would fade away, leaving a simpler and direct visual–object + object–limb configuration. This would be faster, would not compete with other tasks using the object–propositional transformation or the propositional system, and be even less likely to enter awareness (because there are fewer processes involved), but would be less flexible, and subjectively would be focused more on sensory than semantic attributes of the stimuli.

An action schema for drug use might have several eliciting pathways, from each of the three sensory subsystems, any of which could lead to the behavioural outcome independently. An internal change in body state might lead to a cascade from body state to implicational, to propositional, to object, to limb to make a smoker reach for the cigarettes in their pocket, for example; a visual trigger might lead to a simple visual–object + object–limb sequence as the user reaches for the seen stimulus, coupled with a visual–implicational + implicational–somatovisceral sequence to provide the physiological preparation for use. Internal cognitive triggers provided by other thoughts and associations could activate implicational schemata of drug use and trigger the same sort of cascade from implicational to limb as that cued by the change in body state. Longer and more involved patterns of behaviour involving complex task structures stored in propositional and implicational image records could also be automatically activated, although as Tiffany notes, these are less likely to be completely automated.

So far this is just a restatement of Tiffany's theory in a particular framework, and little has been added to his account. What can now be done is to examine the consequences and implications of the patterns of cognitive activity that have been described in ICS. One apparent weakness within Tiffany's theory is the question of how, if craving follows from the controlled inhibition of automatic processes, and those automatic processes can occur without requiring awareness, the controlled inhibition can be initiated. In other words, at what point does the user who is attempting to be abstinent become aware that they are executing an automatic action schema that is leading to drug use, and hence experience craving? The ICS account of Tiffany's theory allows us to examine the ways in which controlled processing might be triggered.

A subjective sense of the self-control of behaviour arises in ICS when implicational and propositional representations are being alternately buffered to bring the individual's motivational/affective state into focal awareness and to select a task structure consistent with the implied goals. During task execution, implicational representations arise from the active propositional representation controlling action, and from the sensory consequences of motor and speech behaviour (as well as from physiological changes in body state). A mismatch between these patterns of implications and the current implicational task schema can lead to an interruption and replanning of behaviour, via an implicational–propositional transformation.

This would allow a user who has the overall personal goal of remaining abstinent to recognise that their own overt behaviour may be leading towards drug use, just as they might notice the behaviour of another person. It also allows them to notice changes in their own physiological state as the schema prepares them for the activity of drug acquisition and the effects of consumption. However, it does not allow the user to notice the internal products of the cognitive processes that are leading to this behaviour. They cannot become implicationally aware of a highly proceduralised visual–object and object–limb sequence, nor of the object and limb representations that are produced, unless those two representations are transformed into implications, and there are no direct processes in ICS to do this. By definition, a proceduralised action schema occurs without requiring focal awareness, and so only the end products of the configuration are available for inspection.

A testable prediction that can be derived from the ICS model, then, is that people could become aware of the implicational representations that are driving changes in their physiological state, if they were engaged in cognitive activity that involved a buffer in the implicational subsystem (e.g., trying to make a qualitative judgement about something, using the implicational–propositional transformation). This is because all information arriving at a subsystem's input array is copied into its image record, and so even information that is not necessarily relevant for the current primary task can enter awareness. This provides the only way in which the thought processes that are part of an automatic action schema could enter awareness before any overt behavioural or physiological change had taken place. The locus of this awareness is the implicational subsystem, and the content of the information that is entering awareness would be psychophysiological in nature because it

is to be used to drive a somatovisceral output. The subjective impression of this trigger for a craving episode would be of a vague feeling of arousal associated with drug acquisition, or a pang of deficit associated with the anticipation of the drug effects.

COMPARING THE TWO ACCOUNTS

In Tiffany's theory and in the EI theory, craving only occurs once the individual becomes aware of some aspect of cognitive activity. The ICS account defines what "becoming aware" consists of in processing terms, and locates the focus of subsequent activity at the implicational level of processing in both accounts. Tiffany's theory limits the nature of the eliciting information to that which has been proceduralised as part of a configuration directed towards producing somatovisceral changes and, due to the nature of proceduralisation, one that is probably triggered by sensory cues. The EI theory allows any activity that might generate the implicational model to result in a craving episode, but the ICS modelling provides a more explicit account of what happens once the implicational schema has been activated and entered awareness. Like Tiffany's theory, the EI model also relies on the idea of proceduralisation or automation of processing to predict why unattended processing tends to travel down well-worn routes, leading to thoughts of substance use. It goes further than Tiffany's theory in detailing the content of the craving episode, especially emphasising the role of mental visual imagery as part of the craving episode, which in ICS terms is a sequence of reciprocal activity involving the implicational, propositional, and object levels of representation.

Tiffany emphasised that his theory allowed for absent-minded lapse in the absence of strong craving, that is, when an abstainer's automated action schemata reached their conclusion without the abstainer noticing their activity and attempting to control their behaviour. The EI theory is in accordance here (although it downplays the role of absent-minded lapses). Neither model expects craving to occur in a situation where the underlying automated cognitive activity does not reach awareness. The ICS models of these theories explain how such absent-minded, automatic activity can occur, by delineating the representations that would have to be involved in the lapse (predominantly visual, object, and limb to control motor behaviour) and those that would have to be heavily involved in a primary task (certainly the propositional and implicational, with no body state involvement).

A key advantage of operationalising the two theories within an information processing account is that it allows the processing steps that each theory requires to be specified, and thus gives an indication of the nature of other cognitive tasks that might interfere with craving, prevent it reaching awareness, or ameliorate its effects once it has occurred. ICS shows that the two theories make different predictions about which processes will inhibit craving. In Tiffany's theory, ICS suggests that craving occurs when implicational representations that are part of an action schema intrude into buffered implicational–propositional processing, or when the user senses their overt or somatovisceral behavioural preparation for drug use. A primary task that requires buffered processing within a different subsystem (e.g., one in which the structure of sounds was in focal awareness), or which avoided the user detecting their preparatory behaviours, would presumably therefore inhibit craving. However, this would only last as long as the user was focused on the inhibiting task. As soon as they stopped attending to it, the craving could resurface. The ICS model of the EI theory suggests that once craving has begun, it could be blocked by preventing the operation of the triad of implicational, propositional, and object subsystems. This could be done most directly by involving the propositional–object and object–propositional transformation processes in another task, e.g., a visual search task, or a visual imagery task. Once this inhibiting task ceases, the cycle of craving would have to be restarted by the generation of another intrusive thought from the antecedents. This might be more likely than before, because the recent substance-related cognitive activity will have left an increased level of activation in relevant transformation processes, but it will not be as likely as suggested by Tiffany's theory.

ASSESSING THE NATURE OF EVERYDAY CRAVINGS

The two theories differ most notably in the role of visual imagery as a key component of elaborated craving: it is central to the EI theory, but not part of Tiffany's theory. The ICS accounts show this to be due to Tiffany's lack of emphasis on what happens during a craving episode. Tiffany's theory, as expressed within ICS, implies that craving episodes would be triggered by the generation of somatovisceral responses to high-level schematic thoughts about a substance, or by an individual noticing their overt behaviour. These should be available for conscious inspection, leading to their attribution as triggering causes of a craving episode. The EI theory does not assume that people have any direct access to the processes that triggered an intrusive thought, and therefore suggests that people may often have little insight these triggers. The EI theory provides a richer account of what follows the trigger. These differences in emphasis between the theories could, in principle, be noticed without the modelling, but we argue that the modelling makes them readily apparent and provides grounded arguments to justify their reality. Once such differences have been noted, then they can be assessed empirically, leading to comparative assessment of the theories.

Tiffany's theory is intended to describe the cravings of people dependent on habit-forming drugs, although it is plausible that the obstruction of action schemata could also cause the weaker cravings experienced by people who habitually use other, non-addictive substances. The EI theory, on the other hand, explicitly defines addictive cravings as the result of the same set of processes that give rise to everyday desires. It is difficult to compare the models on this point, because little empirical work has been carried out into the nature of everyday desires, nor of the cravings for addictive drugs such as alcohol and tobacco by those who are not substance-dependent. We therefore conducted a preliminary survey of everyday cravings using a questionnaire designed to discover more about the subjective aspects of everyday cravings, and to evaluate the differing claims made by the two models.

METHOD

We designed a simple questionnaire and included it in the University of Sheffield's mailing to 1500 new students in September 2002. The questionnaire consisted of two sides of A4, and asked recipients to keep it nearby "until you find that you are craving something". They then had to identify the substance that they were craving by circling one of food, tobacco, alcoholic drink, or soft drink (labelled "non-alcoholic drink" to include tea, coffee, water, etc.), and then specify the substance, and rate the strength of the craving (on a 10-point scale, with the anchors "very slight" and "overwhelming"). There followed a list of 12 potential causes that could have triggered the craving, and 10 statements that could describe the craving (see Table 1). Each had to be rated on a 5-point scale ranging from "not at all" to "definitely" describing the craving. The trigger statements were selected to cover the classes of antecedents identified by the two theories, including bodily sensations, different forms of mental imagery, and intrusive thoughts. The descriptive statements were similarly chosen to contain items that the models suggested should or should not be important.

RESULTS AND DISCUSSION

Within 8 weeks of the mailing (by which time all of the recipients would have moved to Sheffield to start their studies) 361 completed questionnaires

had been received, a response rate of 24%. These replies came from 155 males and 201 females (with 5 not specifying their gender). The median age of the 353 respondents who gave their date of birth was 19 years 8 months (ranging from 14 years 6 months to 55 years 4 months).

Food cravings were reported by 219 people, tobacco cravings by 60, soft drink cravings by 59, and alcoholic drink cravings by 23. The food craving category was broken down by inspecting the specific substance that was reported. This allowed us to identify sub-groups of cravings for chocolate (76 people) and other snacks (75 people), with the remaining (68 people) reporting cravings for main meals, breakfasts, or not specifying any particular substance. The strength of craving scores (reported by 306 people) did not differ significantly between these six craved substance groups, $F(5, 300) = 0.50$, $Mse = 4.14$, ns, with an overall mean of 5.5 and a standard deviation of 2.0 (every point on the 10-point scale was used; the

TABLE 1

Percentage of respondents agreeing with potential trigger and descriptive statements as characterising their craving episode, sorted by mean rating

| Questionnaire items | Theory | Mean rating | Agreement percentage | | | | | χ^2 |
			1	2	3	4	5	
What triggered this craving?								
I suddenly thought about it	E	3.2	15	14	25	26	19	
I felt hungry /thirsty /tired /physical discomfort	Both	3.2	23	13	15	17	31	***
I imagined the smell / taste of it	E	3.1	22	14	20	25	20	**
I pictured myself having it	E	2.8	27	14	26	19	14	
I had nothing else to do / I was bored	T	2.6	36	12	21	18	13	
I saw / heard / smelt it	Both	2.1	61	5	8	14	12	**
Other things I was thinking about reminded me of it	Both	2.0	51	19	13	12	5	
I felt stressed / anxious / sad	E	1.9	59	13	14	9	5	**
I always have it at that time/place	T	1.9	59	13	12	8	9	*
I felt happy	Neither	1.8	55	19	15	8	3	
I was really busy	Neither	1.3	79	11	6	3	1	**
I imagined the sound of myself having it	E	1.3	85	6	6	3	1	
Descriptions of craving episode								
I want it because I am hungry/thirsty/tired/in physical discomfort	Both	3.3	24	8	17	16	34	***
Having it would feel very comforting right now	Both	3.1	18	14	25	24	20	
I am thinking of how much better I will feel after I have had it	Both	3.1	18	15	22	25	20	*
I am imagining the taste of it	Both	3.1	23	12	19	28	18	
I would feel more relaxed if I had it	Both	3.0	22	14	26	21	17	**
I am visualising it	E	2.9	23	15	24	23	15	*
If I don't think about it, my craving will go away	E	2.7	26	21	22	15	16	
I am trying to resist having it	T	2.5	41	14	16	13	17	***
I have it with me right now	Neither	2.0	60	10	10	7	12	**
I can hear myself having it	E	1.4	78	13	5	2	2	

Theory column indicates whether agreement with the item is consistent with the Elaborated Intrusion theory (E), Tiffany's (T), Both, or Neither theories. Agreement ratings range from 1 ("not at all") to 5 ("definitely"). Number of responses per row range between 345 and 356; percentages may not sum to 100 due to rounding. χ^2 tests for each item ($df = 20$; * $p < .05$; ** $p < .01$; *** $p < .001$) indicate contingencies between ratings and craved substance.

mode was 7, used by 81 people, with another 59 using 4, giving a somewhat bimodal distribution). It is notable that the alcohol and tobacco cravings were not significantly stronger than the other cravings, despite the fact that usual levels of cigarette smoking involve significant physical dependence and reported craving. This finding supports the notion that everyday craving for targets other than addictive substances may often be of similar intensity to the levels that are produced by at least the everyday experience of cigarette smoking.

Of the 12 potential triggers, 7 received predominantly low ratings, with more than half of the respondents selecting "not at all" (see Table 1). These include external and internal cueing ("I saw/heard/smelt it" and "Other things I was thinking about reminded me of it"), and negative affective mood ("I was stressed / anxious / sad"), as well as a "habit" statement ("I always have it at that time / place"). One other ("bored") had a modal response of "not at all", but attracted sufficient higher ratings to produce a mean of 2.6 on the 5-point scale, with 52% giving it a rating of 3 or higher. In order of mean rating score, the four triggers that were typically thought to have caused cravings were that the person "suddenly thought about it", "felt ... discomfort", "imagined the taste/smell of it", or "pictured myself having it". The overall picture is that cravers tend not to attribute their thoughts about a substance to any identifiable cue in the environment, but report them as spontaneous (in accordance with the EI theory), or due to somatovisceral sensations (in accord with both theories) and involving olfactory or visual imagery (in accordance with the EI theory). Contrary to Tiffany's theory, cravers do not report experiencing craving in situations where overlearned action schemata might be expected to be activated, such as when they are in habitual usage situations, or when they notice an external or internal cue.

The trigger and descriptive statements all contained response patterns that were highly skewed to one or other end of the 5-point scale for at least one of the substance groups, and so parametric analyses are not suitable. Chi-square tests were therefore used to compare the distribution patterns for each statement to see if there were any differences in response pattern according to craved substance. These showed that of the four highly rated trigger statements, only the ratings for somatovisceral sensations and olfactory imagery differed according to craved substance, with

tobacco cravings being rated as triggered by them *less* often than were soft drinks and the foodstuff cravings (see Figure 3). If the tobacco cravers represent an analogue to a substance-dependent population (which, particularly in the case of nicotine, is not an unreasonable assumption), the ICS model of Tiffany's theory would imply that the opposite pattern should be found, because the physiological changes preparing the person for acquisition and use of tobacco would be more likely to be a trigger for these substances than others. Instead, the somatovisceral sensations and imagery associated with taste and smell are more commonly seen as reasons for craving non-addictive food, snacks, and soft drinks.

The statements describing the cravings generally received higher levels of affirmation than those describing the triggers of the craving. Only two were rated as "not at all" descriptive by more than half of the respondents: "I have it with me right now" and "I can hear myself having it". Four of the five receiving the highest ratings all involve some aspect of physiological relief or reward. The three imagery questions produce markedly different patterns of response: while 65% of respondents rated themselves as "imagining the taste" using 3 or higher, and 61% rated themselves as "visualising it", only 9% rated themselves as "hearing it". Auditory imagery of the craved substance does not seem to play a role, while visual imagery (which might be involved in locating the substance, according to the ICS model of the EI theory) and olfactory imagery (which might be a continuing part of the triggering processing, according to both theories) do emerge as part of everyday cravings.

According to chi-square tests, four statements showed similar patterns of response across all craved substance categories: "Having it would feel very comforting right now", "I am imagining the taste of it", "If I don't think about it, my craving will go away", and "I can hear myself having it". The others produced response patterns that tended to depend on the substance being craved, and suggest that somatovisceral sensations are not as important in tobacco and alcohol craving as in cravings for other substances. "I want it because I am hungry / thirsty / tired / in physical discomfort" was rated 3 or higher less often by the alcohol and tobacco cravers, than by the soft drink and foodstuff groups, with a pattern of responses that was understandably almost identical to that for the equivalent trigger statement. In fact, the modal response for these alcohol and tobacco groups is

'I imagined the smell / taste of it'

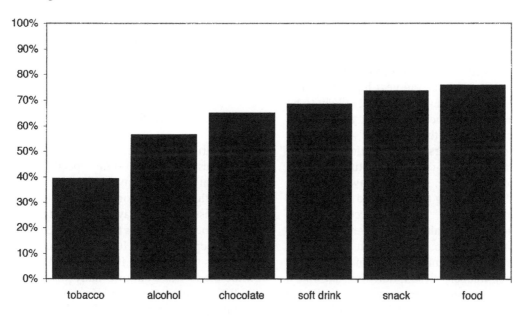

I felt hungry/thirsty/ tired / physical discomfort'

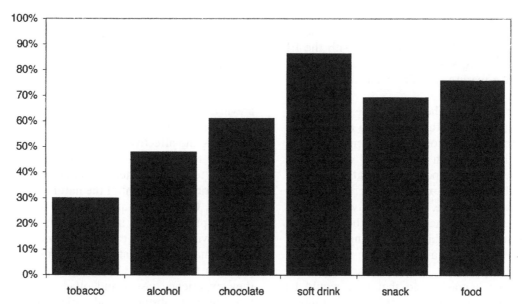

Figure 3. The percentage of responders giving a rating of 3 or above for the somatovisceral imagery and sensation triggers, showing lower affirmation from tobacco and alcohol cravers.

"not at all", but this may be because of the lack of a specific word in the language (and hence in the questionnaire) describing a deficit for nicotine or alcohol, comparable to "hungry" or "thirsty". On the other hand, these two groups clearly have positive expectations about the effect that their substance would have on their affective state:

"I would feel more relaxed if I had it" was rated 3 or higher by 87% of those craving alcohol and 84% craving tobacco. However, "I am thinking of how much better I will feel after I have had it" was only particularly descriptive of those craving a soft drink (34% giving it the top rating of "definitely").

"I am trying to resist having it" was rated highly by 73% of those craving chocolate, and 66% of those craving tobacco, but by only 31% of those in the other substance groups. "I have it with me right now" was only rated highly by tobacco cravers, of whom 28% answered "definitely", almost twice as many as the next highest groups. Perversely, tobacco cravers are highly likely to be trying to resist using their substance, yet are more likely to carry it with them. Tiffany's theory predicts that craving occurs when an action schema is blocked, through self-control or situational factors, yet of our sample, 17 cravers gave a rating of "not at all" for "trying to resist" and "definitely" for "have it with me". Tiffany's account cannot explain these individuals' cravings, yet their mean craving rating was no weaker than that of the whole sample (with a modal value of 7).

The only imagery description that showed a contingency on substance craved was "I am visualising it", and this produced fairly equal ratings in the range 3 or higher of between 54% and 67% for all substances, but with more "definitely" ratings for alcohol, snack, and soft drink cravers, compared to the other groups. The difference here seems to lie in the relative strength of the image, rather than in the presence or absence of visual imagery. This is consistent with the EI claim that craving is equivalent to everyday desire, and is not a feature specific to substance dependence.

It must be stressed here that these descriptions of the triggers and nature of craving episodes are the self-reports of a non-clinical sample. As self-reports, they are open to the usual criticisms of introspective data, especially in that they might reflect what people expect their craving to be caused by or feel like, rather than what craving really does feel like; they might also be influenced by the social desirability of giving particular answers. We tried to avoid these possibilities by asking them to wait until they actually were experiencing a craving, so that they would be more likely to focus on the subjective feelings at that moment, rather than on stereotypical assumptions or expectations, and by allowing the responses to be completely anonymous. Nevertheless, such influences will inevitably remain in investigations into the nature of any subjective phenomenon. The use of a non-clinical sample is partly due to convenience, but it is also influenced by our view that clinical cravings are an extreme form of everyday desires. Those who do not accept this can certainly argue that the craving of an addict is phenomenally different from the cravings that our respondents were experiencing, despite the inclusion of tobacco cravers within our sample. It would indeed be interesting to repeat this kind of study on a substance-dependent population, were a large enough sample available.

CONCLUSION

The information processing approach of ICS has helped us to identify some specific processing steps that could be involved in two models of craving that include cognition as a key explanatory construct for craving. Although Tiffany's theory does not address the subjective content of a craving episode, the ICS model of his theory allows us to infer what this ought to be. Similarly, while the EI theory allows many possible triggers, its ICS model allows us to infer how each of them might operate in practice. For Tiffany's theory, action schemata are primarily proceduralised processes initiated by a sensory representation, and include an implicational–somatovisceral transformation that induces bodily changes preparatory for substance use, which can be detected by a body state–implicational transformation. For the EI theory, the defining character of a craving episode is a reciprocal interaction between the implicational, propositional, and object representations, reflecting the central role of imagery in craving, with the implicational–somatovisceral and body state–implicational transformations providing the affective aspect.

Once these steps were identified, it became possible to evaluate them systematically through an empirical assessment of the nature of everyday cravings. Overall, the questionnaire data suggest that people have little insight into the precursors of a craving episode, reporting them as spontaneous images or somatovisceral sensations that pop into their heads. Once they begin to crave, they experience visual and olfactory images of their desired substance, and anticipate the pleasurable aspects of using it. This is entirely consistent with the EI theory. The modelling of Tiffany's theory is supported by the focus on somatovisceral triggers, but these are reported less strongly by tobacco cravers, which is not what would be expected if Tiffany's account were correct. The data from this sample of non-substance-dependent people is more consistent with the ICS model of the EI theory than with the ICS model of Tiffany's theory.

This study illustrates the benefits of a cognitive account outlined at the start of this paper: by breaking a mental behaviour down into its component parts, we can not only reason about what might be happening during that behaviour, but can examine different speculations about its causes and effects, and devise specific ways of measuring, intervening in, and redirecting mental behaviour. In the case of craving, if further work substantiates the role of imagery, then interventions targeting the same cognitive processes as those necessary for the construction of mental visual imagery could play a role in supporting those attempting to withstand craving for addictive and non-addictive substances.

REFERENCES

Andrade, J., Kavanagh, D. J., & Baddeley, A. D. (1997). Eye movements and visual imagery: A working memory approach to the study of post-traumatic stress disorder. *British Journal of Clinical Psychology, 36*, 209–223.

Baddeley, A. D. (1986). *Working memory*. Oxford: Oxford University Press.

Baddeley, A. D., & Andrade, J. (2000). Working memory and the vividness of imagery. *Journal of Experimental Psychology: General, 129*, 126–145.

Baddeley, A. D., & Hitch, G. (1974). Working memory. In G. A. Bower (Ed.), *Recent advances in learning and motivation* (Vol. 8, pp. 47–89). New York: Academic Press.

Barnard, P. J. (1985). Interacting cognitive subsystems: A psycholinguistic approach to short-term memory. In A. Ellis (Ed.), *Progress in the psychology of language* (Vol. 2, pp. 197–258). Hove, UK: Lawrence Erlbaum Associates Ltd.

Jellinek, E. M. (1960). *The disease concept of alcoholism*. New Brunswick, NJ: Hillhouse Press

Kavanagh, D. J., Andrade, J., & May, J. (2004). *Imaginary relish and exquisite torture: The Elaborated Intrusion Theory of desire*. Manuscript submitted for publication.

Kavanagh, D. J., Freese, S., Andrade, J., & May, J. (2001). Effects of visuospatial tasks on habituation to emotive memories. *British Journal of Clinical Psychology, 40*, 267–280.

Killen, J. D., & Fortmann, S. P. (1997). Craving is associated with smoking relapse: Findings from three prospective studies. *Experimental and Clinical Psychopharmacology, 5*, 137–142.

May, J. (2001). Specifying the central executive may require complexity. In J. Andrade (Ed.), *Working memory in perspective* (pp. 261–277). Hove, UK: Psychology Press.

Monti, P. M., Rohsenow, D. J., Hutchison, K. E., Swift, R. M., Mueller, T. I., Colby, S. M. et al. (1999). Naltrexone's effect on cue-elicited craving among alcoholics in treatment. *Alcoholism: Clinical and Experimental Research, 23*, 1386–1394.

Monti, P. M., Rohsenow, D. J., Swift, R. M., Gulliver, S. B., Colby, S. M., Mueller, T. I. et al. (2001). Naltrexone and cue exposure with coping and communication skills training for alcoholics: Treatment process and 1-year outcomes. *Alcoholism: Clinical And Experimental Research, 25*, 1634–1647.

Norman, D. A. (1981). Categorization of actions slips. *Psychological Review, 88*, 1–15.

O'Malley, S. S., Jaffe, A. J., Chang, G., Rode, S., Schottenfeld, R., Meyer, R. E. et al. (1996). Six-month follow-up of naltrexone and psychotherapy for alcohol dependence. *Archives of General Psychiatry, 53*, 217–224.

O'Malley, S. S., Krishnan-Sarin, S., Farren, C., Sinha, R., & Kreek, M. J. (2002). Naltrexone decreases craving and alcohol self-administration in alcohol-dependent subjects and activates the hypothalamo-pituitary-adrenocortical axis. *Psychopharmacology, 160*, 19–29.

Teasdale, J. D., & Barnard, P. J. (1993) *Affect, cognition and change*. Hove, UK: Lawrence Erlbaum Associates Ltd.

Tiffany, S. T. (1990). A cognitive model of drug urges and drug-use behavior: Role of automatic and non-automatic processes. *Psychological Review, 97*, 147–168.

Wegner, D. M. (1994). Ironic processes in mental control. *Psychological Review, 101*, 34–52.

MEMORY, 2004, *12* (4), 462–466

Individual differences in imagery and reports of aversions

Mark R. Dadds and David Hawes

University of New South Wales, Sydney, Australia

Belinda Schaefer and Kristina Vaka

Griffith University, Brisbane, Australia

Recent theoretical models highlighting the role of imagery in trauma and aversion learning focus on the role of images in memory (e.g., Brewin, Dalgleish, & Joseph, 1996) and images as substitute stimuli in aversive conditioning (Dadds, Bovbjerg, Redd, & Cutmore, 1997). An unanswered question is whether individual differences in imagery are associated with different rates of traumatisation and aversion states (fear and avoidance of various stimuli). We examine one aspect of this: does high imagery ability correlate with the frequency with which people report aversions? Three samples of university students were tested on the Betts Questionnaire Upon Mental Imagery, the Tellegen Absorption Scale, and a new measure we designed to sample of range of aversions. As hypothesised, vividness of imagery showed positive correlations with number of aversions reported. This relationship held after controlling for general neuroticism and proneness to disgust. Results for absorption showed no relationship. The results are unable to disentangle causal paths but suggest a focus on individual differences in imagery vividness may be fruitful for understanding individual differences in aversion learning.

A number of contemporary models of anxiety and trauma assign a role to mental imagery. For example, Brewin, Dalgeish, and Joseph (1996) distinguished between memories for trauma encoded at verbal and sensory-imagery levels, and argued that a preponderance of the latter is associated with persistence of intrusive trauma memories. That is, verbal encoding of memories may allow the person to modify, and thus disempower, frightening memories, whereas memories revolving around sensory images tend to be involuntarily elicited by contextual events and less amenable to conscious modification. Recent studies of this model have provided emerging support for an association between sensory images and the persistence of intrusive memories of unpleasant visual stimuli (Holmes, Brewin, & Hennessy, 2004).

Dadds, Bovbjerg, Redd, and Cutmore (1997) reviewed evidence showing that mental images can substitute for external stimuli in almost all phases of conditioned learning. Typically, the effects of an image are found to be weaker than those of the corresponding actual stimulus; however, imagery can produce strong conditioned responses with important clinical implications (e.g., Jones & Davey, 1990; Redd, Dadds, Bovbjerg, & Taylor, 1993). Some examples of how images can function in conditioning are: imaginal pre-exposure to a stimulus can alter the subsequent orienting response to that stimulus; a mental image of an unconditioned stimulus (e.g., falling from a height) can elicit an unconditioned response; and a mental image of a conditioned stimulus (CS) can elicit a conditioned response.

Correspondence should be sent to Mark R. Dadds, School of Psychology, University of New South Wales, Sydney, Australia 2052. Email: m.dadds@unsw.edu.au

© 2004 Psychology Press Ltd

http://www.tandf.co.uk/journals/pp/09658211.html

DOI: 10.1080/09658210444000070

The evidence reviewed by Dadds et al. (1997) indicates that mental images may facilitate or help overcome various problems of aversive conditioning. The extent that conditioning plays a role in the development and maintenance of common behavioural and emotional problems is mixed and somewhat controversial. Many of the original applications of conditioning theory to clinical problems focused on specific fears (e.g., Wolpe, 1968). While evidence exists that conditioning plays a part in their aetiology, there is convincing evidence that many phobic states are largely unlearned and probably genetically determined to a large extent (e.g., Menzies & Clarke, 1995). Trauma reactions may similarly involve conditioned learning but contemporary models of both trauma and conditioning place far more emphasis on cognitive processing than a simple stimulus-pairing paradigm (e.g., Davey, 1992; Ehlers & Clark, 2000). Learning of medical (e.g., anticipatory nausea and vomiting; Redd, & Andrykowski, 1982) and food aversions are highly compatible with classical conditioning explanations and have particularly strong evidence for a role of imagery in their maintenance (see Dadds et al., 1997; Redd et al., 1993).

Notwithstanding variations in the importance of conditioning in the aetiology of psychological conditions such as phobias, trauma reactions, and food aversions, their treatments share a common focus on exposure as a critical pathway out of the problem. That is, contemporary models of these conditions use in part the idea that the sufferer can benefit from some form of guided exposure to central stimuli (or images of those stimuli) in a way that allows the patient to devalue the threat they pose. Thus, people with many anxious and traumatised conditions function under a cloud of perceived threat in their daily lives, and the most efficacious treatments are those that help the person to face and reinterpret that threat. The extent to which that threat exists and can be modified at the level of imagery is an important question.

Imagery can vary according to state and trait formulations. At least three approaches can be seen in contemporary research. The first studies the content of images as naturalistic phenomena representative of different subject groups. For example, Day, Holmes, and Hackmann (2004 this issue) looked at representative imagery in agoraphobic patients. A second approach manipulates images people hold while engaging in specific tasks and assesses their effects of relevant out-comes. For example, Hirsch, Meynen and Clark (2004 this issue) manipulated the imagery employed by socially phobic persons while undergoing a speaking challenge in order to examine its effects on anxiety. A third approach is to examine the relationship between propensities to imagery as an individual difference related to vulnerability and resilience to emotional and behavioural problems (e.g., Drummond, White, & Ashton, 1978). People differ markedly in the extent to which they are able to generate and manipulate images. Given the putative role of imagery in the development, maintenance, and treatment of emotional and behavioural problems, there should be a relationship between people's proneness to, and skills with, imagery and their mental health.

We developed three alternative hypotheses to test this. The null hypothesis was that there would be no relationship between proneness to, and skills with, imagery and mental health. If this is the case, the importance of imagery may be restricted to its content (e.g., intrusive trauma memories) or it may be an epiphenomenon that is secondary to the psychopathology. Second, high imagery skills might protect against problems by allowing the person skills to manipulate their images so that frightening images can be contained at the benefit of more positive images. Alternatively, high imagery skills might place a person at risk in that frightening images may provide a process by which the person naturally rehearses and inadvertently facilitates their fears. We tested these alternative hypotheses using two aspects of imagery. A traditional measure of imagery, the Betts' Questionnaire Upon Imagery (Sheehan, 1967) assesses a person's ability to generate an image and compare it in vividness to the actual phenomenon. Tellegen's Absorption Scale (Tellegen & Atkinson, 1974) assesses people's ability to absorb themselves in a sensory event. With regard to images, this scale is argued to measure the extent to which a person experiences them as if they are real. To minimise the like-lihood that any relationship observed for imagery was not due to an association with a third variable, we also examined imagery after controlling for measures of general neuroticism and proneness to disgust, both well-known predictors of propensity to learn aversive reactions.

The choice of our measure of "aversions" was more problematic. According to Dadds et al. (1997), images can function to exacerbate a range of specific conditioned reactions. These may involve fear, superstitious avoidance of places, things, and people, and disgust and avoidance reactions to various foodstuffs and organic substances. In order to sample a broad range such reactions, we defined and measured "aversions" loosely, including specific fears, food aversions, and superstitious avoidance of certain stimuli as threatening. Unable to locate such a measure, we developed the Specific Aversion Checklist specifically for this study.

METHOD

Participants

Participants were three samples of undergraduate university students recruited from Griffith University, Australia, across a 4-year period. All received course credit for participation. Sample 1 ($n = 124$) consisted of 79 females and 45 males who ranged in age from 17 to 38 years ($M = 21.6$ years). Sample 2 ($n = 99$) consisted of 76 females and 23 males who ranged in age from 18 to 29 years ($M = 24.0$). Sample 3 ($n = 125$) consisted of 95 females and 30 males who ranged in age from 19 to 32 years ($M = 23.4$ years).

Measures

The Sheehan (1967) revision of the Betts' Questionnaire Upon Imagery (QMI) measures a general ability to imagine across seven sensory modalities (visual, auditory, cutaneous, gustatory, kinaesthetic, olfactory, and organic). Participants are asked to imagine a series of 35 objects and then rate vividness on a 7-point scale. The measure has a long pedigree with excellent psychometric properties. Tellegen's Absorption Scale (TAS) is a 34-item "true–false" questionnaire that measures the participant's ability to become totally involved in sensory events, including imagery. Both original evaluations by Tellegen & Atkinson (1974) and subsequent studies support the psychometric properties of the measure. Neuroticism was measured using Eysenck's Personality Questionnaire-Revised Short Scale (EPQ-N; Eysenck & Eysenck, 1981). Disgust was measured using the Disgust Scale (Haidt, McCauley, & Rozin, 1994), a 32-item scale that measures proneness to disgust across seven domains (food, animals, body products, sex, body violations, death, and hygene) on 3-point Likert

scales. The scale has an internal consistency of .81. The Specific Aversions Checklist (SAC) is an 18-item checklist on which participants check the extent to which they experience an aversion on 5-point Likert scales. The 18 items cover a range of specific fears, aversions to specific foods, drinks, people, and places, and superstitious avoidance of places and things. The SAC can be summed for total number of items checked and mean intensity of items. These correlated at approximately $r = .9$ across the studies and so we only report number of items checked. Evaluations of the internal consistency in the current samples were positive; alpha = .78, .82, and .85 respectively.

Participants completed the questionnaires in small groups of approximately 10 to 20 persons per sitting according to convenience of time scheduling. The order of questionnaire administration varied across samples.

RESULTS

Table 1 shows the correlations between the QMI, TAS, and the aversions SAC across the three samples. In sample 1, both QMI imagery and TAS absorption correlated positively with the SAC, supporting the hypothesis that high imagery skills are associated with increased susceptibility to aversion learning. In sample 2, the correlation between QMI imagery and aversions remains significant after controlling for neuroticism. However, the correlation between TAS absorption and aversions falls to zero once the effects of general neuroticism are controlled. In sample 3, the original zero-order correlations were both zero. However, after controlling for the variance associated with neuroticism and disgust, the correlation between QMI imagery and aversions becomes positive and significant. By contrast, the correlation between absorption and aversions remains at zero.

TABLE 1

Zero-order correlations between imagery, absorption, and the specific aversion on the SAC

	Sample 1	Sample 2	Sample 3
Imagery QMI	.40*	.27* (.19*)[a]	.08 (.24*)[b]
Absorption TAS	.24*	.27* (.05)[a]	.07 (.00)[b]

*$p < .05$; [a] = correlation after controlling for neuroticism; [b] = correlation after controlling for neuroticism and disgust.

DISCUSSION

The results support the hypothesis that certain imagery skills are associated with a vulnerability to learning aversions. Specifically, the ability to create vivid images across a range of sensory modalities was found to be associated with high levels of reported aversions to objects, people, foods, and situations. This association held after controlling for general neuroticism and vulnerability to disgust, and thus imagery is not simply acting as a marker for these more established measures of vulnerability to aversion learning. By contrast, absorption did not show a unique association with aversions. Thus, the findings indicate that there is something specific about the vividness of one's imagery that is associated with aversions, rather than a general propensity to experience sensory events as if they are real.

These results are consistent with Dadds et al.'s (1997) conclusions that ability to form vivid images is associated with enhanced aversive learning. They argued that a mental image can function similarly, albeit more weakly, to a real stimulus in learning to associate innocuous stimuli with threatening, biologically relevant outcomes. The present results do not address specific learning processes. However, they present data about the role of naturally occurring individual differences in imagery and learning. That is, people with highly vivid imagery are more likely to report experiencing a range of aversions to specific stimuli.

Clearly, the current results do not speak to causal direction. Although the conditioning model predicts that vivid imagery leads to aversion learning, a more complex interplay is possible. At the other extreme, it is difficult to see how experiencing aversions could lead to one becoming a more vivid imager—however, the possibility cannot be discounted. Until the processes of learning are more clearly delineated, the exact relationship cannot be known. The image-conditioning model posits a number of potential learning processes. People with high imagery may be primed to seek out threat that is consistent with the content of their mental fears. After experiencing an aversive or traumatic event, high imagers may be more prone to rehearse the unpleasant scenario in a way that escalates or incubates the learning. Consistent with Brewin et al.'s (1996) model, high imagers may be more likely to engage in sensory processing of the event at the expense of more verbal forms of analysis. For other papers looking at the role of imagery in traumatisation,

the reader is referred to Brett and Ostroff (1985) and Laor and Wolmer (2000).

The current results are limited by sole use of undergraduate students and self-report measures. Further, the hypothesised correlation between imagery vividness and aversion was not evident in one of the three samples until general neuroticism had been statistically controlled. The reason for this lack of uniformity across the samples is not known, and replication will be important. Another area that needs further clarification is the construct "aversions". In order to sample a broad range of aversive learning, the checklist developed for this study included a range of items including fears, food aversions, and superstitious avoidance. Although the checklist showed psychometric unity, it may be that treating the items as one may be obscuring more precise relationships. Given that fears, food aversions, and other avoidant behaviour may have multiple and different causal paths, it is unlikely that imagery will function in the same way across problems. Notwithstanding, the current results support the potential utility of studying the role of imagery vividness in a range of behavioural and emotional problems that may involve aversion learning. If imagery vividness is a predictor of vulnerability to such learning, clear clinical and preventive implications abound in terms of identifying people particularly at risk for psychopathology after exposure to trauma in groups likely to be exposed to such events.

REFERENCES

Brett, E. A., & Ostroff, R. (1985). Imagery and post-traumatic stress disorder: An overview. *American Journal of Psychiatry, 142,* 417–424.

Brewin, C. R., Dalgleish, T., & Joseph, S. (1996). A dual representation theory of post-traumatic stress disorder. *Psychological Review, 103,* 670–686.

Dadds, M. R., Bovbjerg, D., Redd, W. H., & Cutmore, T. (1997). Imagery and human classical conditioning. *Psychological Bulletin, 121,* 89–103.

Davey, G. C. L. (1992). Classical conditioning and the acquisition of human fears and phobias: A review and synthesis of the literature. *Advances in Behaviour Research and Therapy, 14,* 29–66.

Day, S. J., Holmes, E. A., & Hackmann, A. (2004). Occurrence of imagery and its link with early memories in agoraphobia. *Memory, 12,* 416–427.

Drummond, P., White, K., & Ashton, R. (1978). Imagery vividness affects habituation rate. *Psychophysiology, 15,* 193–203.

Ehlers, A., & Clark, D. M. (2000). A cognitive model of posttraumatic stress disorder. *Behaviour Research & Therapy, 38,* 319–345.

Eysenck, H. J., & Eysenck, S. B. G. (1981) *Manual of the Eysenck Personality Scales (EPS Adult).* London: Hodder & Stoughton.

Haidt, J., McCauley, C., & Rozin, P. (1994). Individual differences in sensitivity to disgust: A scale sampling seven domains of disgust elicitors. *Personality and Individual Differences, 16,* 701–713.

Hirsch, C. R., Meynen, T., & Clark, D. M. (2004). Negative self-imagery in social anxiety contaminates social interactions. *Memory, 12,* 496–506.

Holmes, E. A., Brewin, C. R., & Hennessy, R. G. (2004). Trauma films, information, and intrusive memory development. *Journal of Experimental Psychology: General, 133,* 3–22.

Jones, T., & Davey, G. C. L. (1990). The effects of cued UCS rehearsal on the retention of differential 'fear' conditioning: An experimental analogue of the worry process. *Behaviour Research and Therapy, 28,* 159–164.

Laor, N., & Wolmer, L. (2000). Image control and posttraumatic symptoms in children following SCUD missile attacks. *Perceptual & Motor Skills, 90,* 1295–1298.

Menzies, R. G., & Clarke, F. C. (1995). The etiology of phobias: A non-associative account. *Clinical Psychology Review, 15,* 23–48.

Redd, W. H., & Andrykowski, M. A. (1982). Behavioral intervention in cancer treatment: Controlling aversive reactions to chemotherapy. *Journal of Consulting and Clinical Psychology, 50,* 1018–1029.

Redd, W. H., Dadds, M. R., Bovbjerg, D., & Taylor, K. (1993). Nausea induced by mental images of chemotherapy. *Cancer, 72,* 629–636.

Sheehan, P. W. (1967) A shortened form of the Betts' Questionnaire Upon Mental Imagery. *Journal of Clinical Psychology, 23,* 386–389.

Tellegen, A., & Atkinson, G. (1974). Openness to absorbing and self-altering experiences ("absorption"); A trait related to hypnotic susceptibility. *Journal of Abnormal Psychology, 83,* 268–277.

Wolpe, J. (1968). *Behaviour therapy.* Stanford, CA: Stanford University Press.

MEMORY, 2004, *12* (4), 467–478

Intrusive and non-intrusive memories in a non-clinical sample: The effects of mood and affect on imagery vividness

Michael Bywaters, Jackie Andrade, and Graham Turpin

University of Sheffield, UK

We studied the number, valence, and vividness of intrusive and non-intrusive memories in two groups (*N* = 20) of pre-screened non-depressed mood and depressed mood undergraduate participants. They were asked to generate as many intrusive memories (IMs) as possible from the prior 2 weeks, together with pleasant and unpleasant non-intrusive memories from the same period. They subsequently formed images of these memories and rated them on measures of vividness, valence, arousal, and overall affect, while having their heart rate, skin conductance, and electromyogram monitored. IMs were common, with participants generating a mean of 1.15 pleasant IMs and 1.60 unpleasant IMs, and there was some evidence that they were mood-congruent. IMs were more vivid than non-intrusive memories, a difference not due to either valence or arousal. We conclude that IMs are a general feature of human memory rather than just a symptom of certain clinical disorders.

The interaction between mood and memory for emotional material has become a well-established basis for theoretical models of depression (see Williams, Watts, McLeod, & Matthews, 1997). Mood-congruent material that has been recently learned, or that forms the basis for autobiographical memories, is selectively recalled according to the individual's mood state. Sometimes mood-congruent memories are spontaneously recalled, intruding into conscious awareness. These "intrusive memories" (IMs) have been most frequently studied in the context of memories of traumatic events associated with post-traumatic stress disorder (Brewin & Holmes, 2003) but also, Brewin and colleagues have reported high levels of IMs in depression. The present study investigated which aspects of emotional events and imagery are associated with the intrusiveness of memories, and tested whether IMs are mood-congruent in non-depressed mood participants as well as in those with depressed mood.

Kuyken and Brewin (1994) interviewed 58 depressed women about their childhood abuse. Of these 58 women, 35 reported experiences meeting the criteria for childhood sexual or physical abuse, and of these 35 women, 30 reported IMs of the abuse in the week prior to the interview. Participants completed the Impact of Events Scale (IES; Horowitz, Wilner, & Alvarez, 1979), obtaining scores equivalent to those of individuals suffering from post-traumatic stress disorder. Higher scores on the IES (both intrusion and avoidance) were related to more severe indices of abuse. Further evidence comes from Spenceley and Jerrom (1997), who compared depressed, recovered, and never-depressed women and found significantly higher levels of intrusion and avoidance of childhood memories among the group of currently depressed women. Brewin, Watson, McCarthy, Hyman, and Dayson (1998) presented further evidence for a link between IMs and the onset of depression. They compared 65 depressed and 65

Correspondence should be sent to Michael Bywaters, c/o Professor Graham Turpin, Department of Psychology, University of Sheffield, Western Bank, Sheffield S10 2TP, UK. Email: bywatm@gosh.nhs.uk

This research was conducted in partial fulfilment of a PhD by the first author at the University of Sheffield and was supported by a bequest from the Lucy Robinson Trust.

DOI: 10.1080/09658210444000089

non-depressed cancer patients matched for age, stage of illness, sex, and type of cancer. The depressed group were divided into severely depressed (those meeting diagnostic criteria) and mildly depressed subgroups; the severely depressed subgroup experienced significantly more IMs than either the moderately depressed group or the control group. In addition, participants in the depressed group were more likely to report that their IMs had either begun concurrently with, or been exacerbated by, the onset of depression.

It would appear that negative IMs in clinical samples are associated with the severity and possible onset of depression. However, little is known about the relationship between IMs and affect in non-clinical samples, despite IMs being common. In Brewin, Christodoulides, and Hutchinson's (1996) study of 76 students, all participants reported at least five intrusive images in the previous 2 weeks. In addition, Berntsen has also found evidence of both pleasant and unpleasant intrusive memories in non-clinical samples (e.g., Berntsen, 1996, 2001). Berntsen argues that it is the "intensity" of the memories that leads them to become intrusive, rather than the valence of the memory.

The present study therefore explored the relationship between current mood state and frequency, valence, and vividness of recent IMs in non-clinical participants selected as experiencing either depressed or non-depressed mood. Neither Brewin et al. (1996), nor Berntsen (1996, 2001) measured the mood of participants, and therefore it is unknown whether non-clinical IMs are mood-congruent. Given the general finding that autobiographical memories are easier to retrieve when mood-congruent (Williams et al., 1997), we predicted that IMs would also be mood-congruent, hence people with depressed mood would experience predominantly negative intrusions and those with non-depressed mood would have more positive intrusions.

Given the findings discussed earlier, of higher rates of intrusion in more depressed patients, we also predicted an association between the frequency of IMs and the extremes of valence of the memories: highly pleasant and highly unpleasant memories would both be highly salient and therefore more likely to intrude than less emotive memories. In other words, IMs may simply be a subset of autobiographical memories that are readily triggered because they are congruent with currently activated schemata and are exception-

ally salient (that is, exceptionally vivid, arousing, and emotive).

We previously conducted an experiment using pictorial stimuli selected from the International Affective Picture System (IAPS; Lang, Öhman, & Vaitl, 1988). The IAPS stimuli have been extensively rated and have normative values for valence (pleasantness) and arousal levels, and thus we chose a range of visual stimuli, spanning pleasant to unpleasant, and highly arousing to neutral. We found that mental images of emotive (pleasant *or* unpleasant) scenes are more vivid than images of neutral stimuli (Bywaters, Andrade, & Turpin, 2004 this issue). We were therefore interested in replicating this finding with autobiographical memories and testing whether vividness of recollections was related to their tendency to intrude. To do this, we compared participants' ratings of the vividness, valence, arousal, and overall affect of IMs with their ratings of non-intrusive pleasant and unpleasant memories from the same period. We predicted that intrusive memories would be mood-congruent. We also predicted that mood-congruent images would be more vivid than those images that were not mood-congruent. We hypothesised that intrusive memories would be more vivid than non-intrusive memories, and that depressed mood participants would have more frequent intrusions than non-depressed mood participants (based on the findings of Brewin et al., 1998).

We also obtained several psychophysiological variables: Specifically, we measured skin conductance (SC), and facial electromyography (EMG) and heart rate (HR), as indices of arousal and valence respectively (see Lang, Bradley, & Cuthbert, 1998; Lang, Greenwald, Bradley, & Hamm, 1993). We predicted that participants would show greater skin conductance responses when forming images of the IMs, indicating increased arousal. We predicted that EMG would act as an objective measure, indicating whether differences in vividness between IMs and non-IMs were due solely to differences in valence. Holmes, Brewin, and Hennessy (2004) had reported a recent finding of a reduction in heart rate during participants' "intrusion sequences" (points during a traumatic film that subsequently intruded). In addition, we were interested to see if this reduction also occurred during the imaging of IMs, and if this HR reduction did occur, whether it occurred for all intrusive imagery or solely negative intrusive imagery.

METHOD

Participants

Potential undergraduate participants from the Department of Psychology in Sheffield were screened using the Beck Depression Inventory (BDI). To derive depressed mood and non-depressed mood groups, students whose BDI scores were either 3 or below, or 9 or above were then contacted via email and asked to participate in the study either in return for a payment of £5 or for course credits; participation was entirely voluntary. Nine participants were excluded from the study as their scores had fallen outside the cut-off points by the day of the study. Two groups ($N = 20$) were determined based on their final mood scores; those with a BDI score of 3 or below (mean $= 1.4$, $SD = 1.10$), and those with a score of 9 or above (mean $= 13.7$, $SD = 4.47$). Of these participants, 34 were female and 6 were male, with ages ranging from 18 to 50 (mean $= 21$ years and 4 months).

With respect to the cut-offs employed, Cox, Enns, Borger, and Parker (1999) compared analogue and clinical samples based on the phenomenology of their depressive experience, using a cut-off of above and below 9 on the BDI. They concluded that the differences found between their samples were of a quantitative rather than qualitative nature. Analysis indicated that the symptom structure of the analogue and clinical samples was very similar, differing only in severity. We therefore used a BDI score of 9 or above as our measure of depressed mood, (an analogue sample for depression), as compared with a non-depressed mood/neutral mood group of participants with BDI scores of 3 or below. Since we did not specifically measure positive hedonic tone, we can only describe this group as lacking depressive mood as measured by the BDI.

Apparatus

The study was conducted within a psycho-physiology laboratory, which comprised two adjoining sound-attenuated rooms (3.6 m × 2.6 m) linked via a two-way intercom (model MIC 404): one room for testing and the other for data acquisition. Participants sat in a semi-reclining Parker-Knoll chair approximately 90 cm away from the screen, which was positioned at eye level. Ratings of valence and arousal were obtained using a computerised version of the Self-Assessment Mannequin (SAM), a schematic representation of the feelings of valence and arousal, used to rate the IAPS slides (e.g., Lang et al., 1993). Vividness was recorded using an 11-point computer-based vividness scale (Andrade, Kavanagh, & Baddeley, 1997).

Bipolar recording of skin conductance was obtained using two domed SLE (Ag-AgCl) 9 mm electrodes attached with adhesive collars (19.6 mm^2) to the palmar surface of the medial phalanx of the first and second fingers from the non-preferred hand. A purpose-made gel (0.05m NaCl in a methyl cellulose base) was used as an electrolyte (Grey & Smith, 1984; although see Clements, 1989). A Biopac GSR100A pre-amplifier with a sensitivity setting of 10 μmhos and a constant voltage (0.5 v) was employed.

Heart rate was measured using two stainless steel plate electrodes (6 × 4 cm) strapped to the lower arms using a commercial ECG electrode gel (Dracard) as the electrolyte. A Biopac ECG100A was used to measure the R-wave of the ECG using a sensitivity setting between 10 and 20 mV.

The facial EMG data were collected from the zygomaticus major and the corrugator supercilli muscles using two domed SLE (Ag-AgCl) 9 mm electrodes attached with adhesive collars. The electrode sites were prepared and positioned as suggested by Fridlund and Cacioppo (1986). Signals were integrated online using a Biopac EMG100 integrator and consisted of full wave rectification, followed by a 10 Hz low pass filter.

The preamplifiers were connected to a MP100 D/A converter and optically isolated between the participant and a Apple Macintosh 6100/66 computer employed to analyse the data using the "AcqKnowledge version 3.1" software.

Procedure

Participants were informed that they were taking part in an experiment exploring the relationship between imagery vividness and memory. They gave written consent. They were then read the following definition, and asked to describe the most frequent intrusive memory that they had experienced in the previous 2 weeks (Brewin et al., 1996, p. 108):

> Intrusive memories are memories of a specific event or incident that has happened to you sometime previously. They can be pleasant (positive) or unpleasant (negative) memories that

interrupt day to day activity and may be difficult to control. Some of these memories may be hard to mention or even embarrassing. It is important nevertheless that you are as honest as possible if the research is to be of value.

Participants were also asked how long ago was the incident leading to the intrusive memory, and gave an estimate of the number of times the image had intruded in the prior 2 weeks. They were then asked to think of and describe one pleasant and one unpleasant memory that had not intruded in the previous 2 weeks. They were given the following instructions to help generate these memories:

Please think of a memory from roughly around the same time period as [their first intrusive memory], that is a pleasant (positive) memory [or unpleasant (negative) memory]. This should be a memory of a specific event that has NOT interrupted your day to day activities in the past two weeks, and that you do not have difficulty controlling.

This procedure was repeated with the next most frequent intrusive memory, and equivalent non-intrusive memories, and continued until participants reported no more IMs. The three most frequent memories, and their corresponding three pleasant and three unpleasant non-IMs, were used for the imagery phase of the experiment. If participants could not generate three IMs from the previous 2 weeks, they were asked to describe a memory that had intruded at some point in their lives, matched with a pleasant and unpleasant memory from roughly the same time. These memories were then used in the imagery phase to ensure that every participant had the same imagery procedure, recalling three IMs, and three pleasant and three unpleasant non-intrusive memories. We recorded how long it took participants to generate these memories.

Participants also completed a shortened version of the Eysenck Personality Questionnaire (EPQ; Eysenck & Eysenck, 1969), the Spielberger State-Trait Anxiety Inventory (STAI; Spielberger, Gorsuch, Lushene, Vagg, & Jacobs, 1977), the shortened version of the Betts' Questionnaire upon Mental Imagery (QMI; Sheehan, 1967), and the intrusion subscale from the Impact of Events Scale (IES; Horowitz et al., 1979), which could refer to either pleasant or unpleasant images.

While participants were completing the questionnaires, the experimenter typed text prompts for the participants' memories into a PsyScope script, which then randomly cued the participant's imagery in the next phase of the experiment. Participants were then prepared for the psychophysiology recordings of heart rate, skin conductance, and facial electromyography (zygomaticus major and corrugator supercilli).

A second set of instructions was presented for 15 seconds, followed by a 3-minute period of recording psychophysiological baseline data, after which the imagery phase began. For 6 seconds, participants viewed a description of a memory, either one of their own IMs, or one of their non-intrusive autobiographical memories. When the description disappeared from the screen, participants closed their eyes for 6 seconds and tried to form as vivid an image of the memory as possible. A tone cued participants to open their eyes, and they were asked to rate their imagery for vividness, from 0 (no image at all) to 10 (image as clear and vivid as normal vision), overall emotion, from −10 (extremely negative), through 0 to +10 (extremely positive). Participants were also given 15 seconds to rate their emotional response to the image on the computerised version of the SAMs rating scales (measuring arousal and valence). Following each trial, participants viewed a screen asking them to relax, which was presented for 18–30 seconds, before the next trail began again. Participants completed a total of nine trials in the imagery phase (three IMs, three pleasant, and three unpleasant non-intrusive memories), with stimuli being presented in a random order for each participant. Psychophysiological recordings were taken throughout each phase of the experiment, and quantified off-line following completion of the experiment. Upon completion of the experimental tasks, the physiological transducers were removed and participants were thanked and debriefed as to the nature of the study.

RESULTS

First we report the frequency of IMs, then we present detailed analyses of the effects of mood and memory types on ratings of valence, arousal, vividness, and strength of emotion. Finally, psychophysiological responding during the recall of IMs and other memories will be examined. Participants were asked to generate other, previously intrusive memories during the experiment if they had fewer than three IMs from the prior 2 weeks. However, this was to ensure that each participant completed the same procedure of rating nine memories. Only those memories identified as intrusive in the two weeks prior to the experiment were analysed and reported as intrusive memories in the results section.

Self-report data

Participants' self-report data were reduced as follows: The mean was calculated for each participant's rating of vividness, valence, arousal, and overall emotion, for each of the memory types (IM, pleasant memory, and unpleasant memory). Averages were also calculated for participants' frequency, latency, and IES scores, by finding the mean of these scores for their three IMs. These data will be the data used in the results section unless otherwise specified. However, in the interview phase of testing, participants were encouraged to generate as many IMs as they could, and some additional analyses employed the total number of IMs generated—for these the complete data are used.

Number, frequency, and type of intrusive memories

The first issue addressed is whether intrusive memories are predominantly negative, regardless of mood, or whether they are mood-congruent. Participants rated each of their intrusive memories on a scale of pleasantness, ranging from highly pleasant, to highly unpleasant. Using these ratings of the IMs' valence, we were able to categorise them as either pleasant or unpleasant. The mean number of IMs generated was 2.75, with participants generating a mean of 1.15 pleasant IMs and 1.60 unpleasant IMs. The range of IMs generated was between 1 and 5, with only one participant generating 5 IMs.

The secondary prediction based on Brewin's work was that depressed mood participants would have more frequent intrusions (i.e., the same memory intruding more often) than non-depressed mood participants. This was found to be the case, with depressed mood participants experiencing significantly more frequent intrusions, $t(1, 38) = 3.71, p < .01$.

We hypothesised that IMs would be mood-congruent. We suggested that participants with depressed mood (high BDI score) would report predominantly negative IMs, whereas those with higher mood would report predominantly positive

IMs. This prediction was supported, with depressed mood participants having a significantly greater number of negative intrusive memories, $t(1, 38) = 2.95, p < .01$, and non-depressed mood participants having a significantly greater number of pleasant intrusive memories, $t(1, 38) = 2.67, p < .05$. Finally, the groups were compared on the total number of intrusions experienced, with no significant difference found, $t(1, 38) = 1.57, p = .12$.

Comparisons of intrusive and non-intrusive memories

We speculated that, if IMs were indeed mood-congruent, they might simply represent a particularly vivid, extremely valenced, and highly arousing subset of normal autobiographical memories. We therefore compared ratings of IMs with ratings of pleasant and unpleasant non-intrusive memories across the depressed mood and non-depressed mood groups. Mixed measures ANOVA was used, with memory type as the within-subjects factor and mood (depressed mood or non-depressed mood) as the between-subjects factor.

Imagery vividness showed a main effect of memory type, $F(2, 76) = 11.97, p < .001$. Planned comparisons revealed that all of the memory types differed from one another, with IMs being most vivid, pleasant memories being next most vivid, and unpleasant memories being least vivid (see Figure 1). Participants' mood did not affect vividness $(F < 1)$, and the interaction between

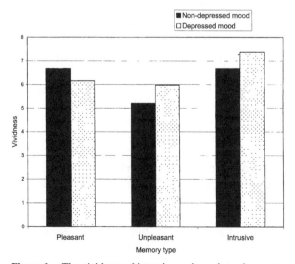

Figure 1. The vividness of intrusive and non-intrusive memories for depressed mood and non-depressed mood groups.

mood and memory type marginally failed to reach significance, $F(2, 76) = 3.010$, $p = .051$.

This finding that IMs were more vivid than negative, non-intrusive memories could reflect a difference in the arousal or valence of the images being generated. In a prior experiment by Bywaters et al. (2004 this issue), extremely valenced images and highly arousing images were shown to be more vivid than more neutral images, and it is possible that the differences in vividness were due to corresponding differences in the arousal and valence of the memories. However, mixed measures ANOVA showed that arousal ratings were not affected by memory type, $F(2, 74) = 1.28$, $p = .29$, or mood ($F < 1$), and the interaction between memory type and mood was not significant, $F(2, 74) = 2.01$, $p = .10$.

To compare the valence of the different memory types, it was necessary to recode the valence scores to give a measure of strength rather than direction of emotion. "Emotional magnitude scores" were therefore generated by converting the SAM scores to numbers (1 = highly pleasant, 9 = highly unpleasant) and calculating the distance of each score from the mid-point (5). These scores were then averaged by memory type as explained above. Then these scores were subjected to mixed measures ANOVA as above. This revealed a significant main effect of memory type, $F(2, 78) = 8.56$, $p < .001$, but planned comparisons showed that although the IMs and pleasant memories differed from the unpleasant memories, they did not differ from each other. Thus the finding that the IMs were more vivid than the pleasant memories cannot be attributed to a difference in pleasantness or arousal, as these are equivalent for the pleasant and IM memory types. This suggests that something else is mediating the vividness of the IMs, but not the non-intrusive memories. Given that the interaction between mood and memory type for the vividness scores was so close to significance, more detailed analyses are required to further investigate whether mood congruence is this mediating factor. These are reported below.

Comparisons of pleasant and unpleasant IMs

As explained above, the IMs used in the aforementioned ANOVAs included both pleasant and unpleasant IMs within the IM category. Therefore, the IMs were separated using the participant's own rating of the memory into "pleasant

IMs" and "unpleasant IMs", to test whether unpleasant IMs are more vivid than pleasant IMs and whether this relationship is mediated by mood. Mean vividness, valence, and arousal scores were then calculated as above for each IM category for each person. Not all participants generated both pleasant and unpleasant intrusions, hence the numbers for each analysis differ: 33 participants were included for the unpleasant IMs whereas only 28 were included in the case of the pleasant IMs. A mixed ANOVA revealed that the pleasant IMs were more vivid than the unpleasant IMs, $F(1, 19) = 8.69$, $p < .01$. In addition, the depressed mood participants reported more vivid imagery than the non-depressed mood participants, $F(1, 19) = 5.65$, $p < .05$. There was no interaction between mood and IM type ($F < 1$). These results are displayed in Figure 2.

Emotional magnitude scores were calculated for pleasant and unpleasant IMs. Pleasant IMs were more emotive than negative IMs, $t(22) = 2.08$, $p < .05$. Thus the difference in vividness scores between the pleasant and unpleasant IMs may be due to the difference in emotional magnitude.

Comparison of IMs with non-intrusive memories

For the unpleasant memories, mixed measures ANOVA showed that IMs were more vivid than non-intrusive memories, $F(1, 31) = 6.12$, $p < .05$. Depressed mood participants reported more vivid

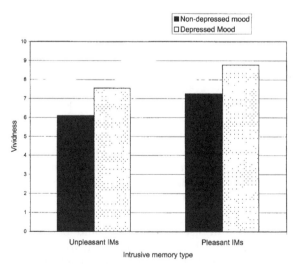

Figure 2. The vividness of pleasant and unpleasant intrusive memories for depressed mood and non-depressed mood groups.

imagery than non-depressed mood participants, $F(1, 31) = 6.76, p < .05$, but this effect of mood did not interact with that of memory type ($F < 1$). A t-test of the valence scores for unpleasant memories revealed that IMs were more unpleasant than the non-intrusive memories, $t(32) = 2.06, p < .05$. This difference in valence might explain the difference in vividness of the unpleasant intrusive and non-intrusive memories.

For the pleasant memories, IMs were more vivid than non-intrusive memories, $F(1, 26) = 14.54, p < .001$, and there was no effect of mood on vividness ($F < 1$). However, there was an interaction between mood and intrusiveness, $F(1, 26) = 4.43, p < .05$, such that the depressed mood group had more vivid imagery for pleasant IMs than the non-depressed mood group, whereas the non-depressed mood group had more vivid imagery for the pleasant non-intrusive memories. For the pleasant memories, the difference in vividness between IMs and non-IMs could not be explained in terms of valence, which was similar for both memory types, $t(28) = 1.25, p = .22$. This replicates the main initial finding that these intrusive memories were more vivid than their non-intrusive counterparts, and also that this cannot be explained by an equivalent difference in valence.

Psychophysiology results

Heart rate

The heart rate data were quantified offline and inter-beat intervals were calculated from each R-wave. These were then further transformed to second by second data using a purpose written program (Turpin & Siddle, 1989). The 12 seconds immediately prior to a memory cue were taken as a baseline measure, and the 6 seconds of viewing the memory cue, and the 6 seconds of imagery were quantified. Baseline data were analysed using ANOVA but no significant main effects or interactions were found that suggest that the groups were equivalent, $Fs < 1.68, p > .05$.

Text reading and imagery. The baseline for each memory was subtracted from each second of text viewing. A mean profile score for each memory type was then derived by averaging across the three memories within a memory type. There was no significant main effect of memory type, $F(2, 76) = 0.836, p = .58$, or of mood, $F(1, 38) = 0.052, p = .89$. There was, however, a significant main effect of seconds, $F(5, 190) = 10.721, p < .001$,

which indicates reliable heart rate responding. Tukey's HSD post-hoc analyses revealed that there was significantly deceleration over the first 3 seconds when compared with acceleration over the fourth, fifth, and sixth seconds. All higher-order interactions with seconds were non-significant ($Fs < 0.144, p > .05$) with the exception of a significant interaction between memory type and seconds, $F(10, 380) = 1.88, p < .05$. The interaction is due to a relatively larger acceleration for intrusive memories over seconds three and four, as compared with pleasant and unpleasant non-intrusive memories. These data are shown in Figure 3. Further analysis of the interaction is presented below.

The imagery data were analysed in the same way as for the text reading data. There was a significant interaction only between memory type and mood group, $F(2, 76) = 4.335, p < .05$, which indicated higher heart rates for the neutral mood participants when imaging intrusive memories, as compared with little change in the depressed mood group. All other main effects and interactions were nonsignificant ($Fs < 1.77, p > .05$).

Pleasant and unpleasant intrusive memories. Following the analysis of the self-report data above, pleasant and unpleasant memories were separated and HR profiles were again calculated. These analyses revealed reliable heart rate profiles within the text reading, $F(5, 125) = 2.51, p < .05$, but no other main effects or interactions were significant for either text reading or imagery ($Fs < 2.01, p > .05$). Similarly no significant main effects or interactions were obtained for the HR imagery data ($Fs < 3.17, p > .05$). Overall the HR results suggest that intrusive memories differ in affective response from non-intrusive memories, which appear to be equivalent.

Skin conductance responses

Viewing and imagery. Skin conductance data were analysed in the same fashion as Lang et al. (1993). The conductance response magnitude (μsiemens) was measured for each stimulus, and taken as the largest response between 0.9 s and 4 s after either text cue presentation or imagery commencement. The baseline at text or imagery onset was then subtracted from this SC value, thus giving a skin conductance level change score. As these data were positively skewed, log transformations were used to normalise the data [log (SCR+1)]. These scores were then averaged by

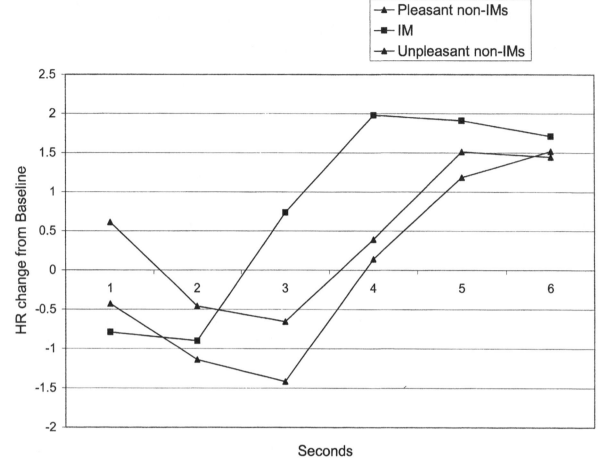

Figure 3.   Heart rate when reading cues for different memory types, by seconds.

memory type, giving one score per memory type, per person.

The only significant effect for skin conductance was an effect for mood within the text viewing phase, $F(1, 38) = 4.98$, $p < .05$. Tukey's HSD calculations reveal that this difference was due to the depressed mood group having significantly greater SCL values than the nondepressed mood group. All other effects were nonsignificant for either phase ($Fs < .72$, $p > .05$). These findings are consistent with the lack of self-reported differences in arousal across the memory conditions.

Pleasant and unpleasant intrusive memories. Again as above, these two types of intrusive memory were separated and compared. One-within, one-between ANOVAs were conduced, with intrusive memory valence and mood group as the factors. No significant effects were obtained for any of these analyses ($Fs < 3.95$, $p > .05$).

EMG data

The EMG data from both the corrugator and zygomatic muscles were also averaged second by second for the 6 seconds of text reading and the 6 seconds of imagery. A baseline of the score for the 12 seconds immediately prior to text presentation for each stimulus was taken and subtracted from each successive second to give EMG change scores. These change scores were then averaged by memory type.

Viewing and imagery. ANOVAs were conducted as above, with memory type and seconds as the within-participants factors, and mood group as the between-participants factor. No significant effects or interactions for either the viewing or imagery phases were obtained for the corrugator muscle ($Fs < 1.02$, $p > .05$). However, there was a significant main effect of memory type on the viewing data, $F(2, 76) = 6.46$, $p < .01$, for the zygomatic muscle. This difference was due to significantly greater responses for intrusive memories when compared with pleasant memories. There was also a significant interaction between memory type and seconds, $F(10, 380) = 2.18, p < .05$.

All other interactions were nonsignificant ($Fs < 1.02, p > .05$). The imagery data for the zygomatic muscle also revealed a significant effect of memory type, $F(2, 76) = 5.97, p < .01$, but no other effects were significant ($Fs < 2.39, p > .05$).

Pleasant and unpleasant intrusive memories. As before, the intrusive memories were separated into pleasant intrusive memories and unpleasant intrusive memories and analysed using a 2-within, 1-between ANOVA. For both the text viewing and imagery data for the corrugator muscle, there were no significant effects ($Fs < 3.78, p > .05$). Similarly there were no effects for the zygomatic muscle viewing phase ($Fs < 1.94, p > .05$). However, there was a main effect of seconds, $F(5, 125) = 2.31, p < .05$, for the zygomatic imagery phase that indicated a general increase in response over time. No other effects were significant ($Fs < 1.37, p > .05$).

DISCUSSION

We compared the intrusive and non-intrusive memories of relatively depressed mood and non-depressed mood undergraduate participants. We replicated Brewin et al.'s (1996) results with an unselected undergraduate sample by showing that IMs are relatively common even in a non-clinical sample, although they were somewhat less common in our sample than in Brewin et al.'s original study. We extended their study by showing that, for our sample, IMs tended to be unpleasant and that intrusions were experienced more often by depressed mood than by non-depressed mood participants. However pleasant IMs were rated as more extremely valenced and more vivid than the unpleasant IMs. This is further evidence that IMs are not necessarily negative and are not peculiar to disorders such as depression and PTSD. Rather, they appear to be a general feature of memory.

We found some evidence to support our prediction that IMs are mood-congruent, with depressed mood being associated with a higher number of unpleasant IMs and non-depressed mood being associated with a higher number of pleasant IMs. In this sense, IMs are like other autobiographical memories (see Williams et al.,

1997). There was also a tendency for depressed mood participants to report more vivid imagery for intrusive memories—replicating the findings of Bywaters et al. (2004 this issue)—but for non-depressed mood participants to have more vivid pleasant non-intrusive memories. Baddeley and Andrade (2000) found that image vividness is partially contingent upon the ease of accessibility of information related to the image in long-term memory (LTM). Thus the tendency of memory vividness to be mood-congruent supports the general claim that current mood state affects accessibility of information in long-term memory.

We predicted that IMs would be more vivid, arousing, and more extremely valenced (i.e., more strongly pleasant or unpleasant) than non-intrusive memories. We found that IMs were indeed more vivid than non-IMs, but not more arousing. The valence data were somewhat inconsistent—thus the unpleasant IMs were more vivid and more unpleasant than the unpleasant non-IMs, and the pleasant IMs were more vivid but no more pleasant than the pleasant non-IMs. This inconsistency suggests that valence alone is insufficient to explain the tendency of IMs to be more vivid than non-intrusive autobiographical memories. Given the finding that IMs are particularly vivid, and Baddeley and Andrade's (2000) argument that vivid memories are those that are particularly accessible in LTM, we are forced to conclude that IMs are vivid because they are very easily and frequently recalled. Further research is needed to address the issue of what makes recall so easy for some memories that they are recalled apparently spontaneously and uncontrollably. The present study has established that this ease of recall is not an inevitable feature of arousing and extremely valenced memories.

Psychophysiological measures

The pattern of responding for HR, SC, and EMG was consistent with previous studies of imagery (Witvliet & Vrana, 1995). Interestingly the overall response to text cued recall of intrusive memories was an initial heart rate deceleration followed by a subsequent acceleration. This is similar to the profile reported by Holmes et al. (2004) and suggests that greater attention is being devoted to the intrusive image (Cook & Turpin, 1997). The major psychophysiological differences that were obtained corresponded to greater activity for both HR acceleration and zygomotor EMG for intrusive memories compared to non-intrusive ones. Increased physiological arousal might also be an additional distinctive factor associated with self-reported vividness, which characterises intrusive memories. The lack of skin conductance response differences was perhaps not surprising given the fact that the memories had not been rated differently according to their arousing properties. Similarly, the lack of differences for corrugator EMG may reflect that participants were instructed to close their eyes when imaging.

Limitations

While the results of this study have implications for the theoretical understanding of IMs, the findings should be interpreted with some caution. First, the reported number of intrusive memories experienced in the 2 weeks prior to the experiment, and the frequency of those intrusions, were assessed retrospectively. This leaves the possibility of inaccurate estimates of IMs. There is also evidence of a mood-congruent recall effect, making it more likely that the memories recalled at the time of experiment would be biased to fit the hypotheses (i.e., that the depressed mood group would recall more negative memories and vice versa). In addition, albeit anecdotally, participants did find the task of recalling intrusive memories difficult, and suggested that they were unable to bring all of their IMs to mind when asked to recall them. Although the procedure here was the same as Brewin et al. (1996), and participants were given as much time as they desired (including prompting to continue thinking where appropriate), it may be that participants had more IMs but were simply unable to recall them at the time of the experiment. In future, a design that involves participants keeping a diary of intrusive memories and the frequency of intrusions may lead to a more accurate measure of IMs.

The second reason for caution in generalising from this study is that, by design, it was conducted with a non-clinical sample. Although this population is interesting to investigate, it may be that the intrusions in a depressed mood group are qualitatively different from those in a depressed sample. There is evidence to suggest that the negative affect experienced in depressed mood is qualitatively similar to that experienced in clinical depression, differing only in severity (e.g., see Cox et al., 1999). However this is a far from universal view of the depressive experience: There are others who argue for a distinct difference between the experiences of those who are depressed and those who are not (e.g., Coyne, 1994). Whilst the evidence from Cox et al. (1999) is persuasive, no one has looked explicitly at the *qualitative* nature of intrusive memories in depression, nor compared the qualitative experience of IMs in depression with IMs from a non-clinical sample.

A related limitation stems from what Brewin and colleagues call the "here and now" element of intrusive memories. In this experiment, participants were asked to recall memories that had previously intruded, therefore the memories were being brought to mind in an effortful fashion, rather than forcing their way into consciousness. Thus the images being rated for vividness were memories *that had been intrusive in the past*, rather than being intrusive at the time. This is especially important given that, particularly in intrusions in PTSD, Brewin (Brewin, Dalgleish, & Joseph, 1996) posits two different mechanisms for memory retrieval; one being effortful and able to be retrieved at will (verbally accessible memories; VAMs), and the other being intrusive and only accessible in an automatic fashion (situationally accessible memories; SAMs). Therefore, it is possible that the mechanisms underlying the intrusions were not being activated during the imagery task. Nonetheless, given that participants were possibly accessing the supposedly "weaker" VAMs, it is even more impressive that they were rated as being significantly more vivid than the non-intrusive emotionally charged memories. If, as is suggested above, there was no difference between the effortfully remembered "non-intrusive memories" and the effortfully remembered "intrusive memories", one would expect no differences in vividness (particularly once valence and arousal had been factored out). Thus it seems that even though these memories might not have been intrusive during the experiment, they still have a different phenomenological impact even when they are effortfully recalled.

A related issue is that although only those memories that had intruded in the prior 2 weeks were included in the analysis as intrusive memories, some of the "non-intrusive memories" may have been intrusive in the past. Therefore, instructions asking for memories that had never been intrusive would have been a clearer request for non-intrusive memories.

Another issue raised as a product of conducting this experiment is the need to tighten the definition of "intrusive memories/imagery".

Anecdotally, several people asked during the experiment whether the images had to be memories, or whether they could be images that had intruded, but which had not actually happened. In terms of the verbal modality, this distinction is the same as between ruminating about *past* events, as opposed to worrying about potential negative *future* events. In this experiment, participants were only allowed to use memories of events that had actually happened. However, there may be differences between intrusive images that rely on actually experienced events (on which our hypotheses were based), and those that have not happened (possibly similar to the negative thoughts about the future in Beck's cognitive triad).

Finally, this study only considered "internal" aspects of memories. The limited time span from which memories were recalled probably minimises the effects of "external" factors on recall. To some extent, the intrusive memories we elicited were a feature of the environmental factors that pertained in the 2 weeks prior to the study. Had these external factors differed, for example if participants had been on vacation rather than at university, then different memories might have intruded. In other words, for a memory to become intrusive may require not only that the memory is mood-congruent, arousing, and highly pleasant or unpleasant, but also that there are appropriate retrieval cues in the environment. It is conceivable that altered attentional focus in conditions like PTSD and depression (see Williams et al., 1997) leads to repeated exposure to retrieval cues for negative memories, and that repeated retrieval of those memories in turn enhances their accessibility, until they are recalled so automatically that they are immune to conscious control and are experienced as intrusions.

CONCLUSIONS

In conclusion, while the results of this experiment need to be regarded with some caution, they shed some light on the nature of intrusive memories. We have established that IMs in a non-clinical sample are common, frequently pleasant rather than unpleasant, and that they are more vivid than equally valenced and arousing non-intrusive memories. Psychophysiological data would also suggest that IMs are associated with greater physiological arousal in the form of greater heart rate accelerations and zygomotor EMG. We found

some evidence, albeit quite weak, for IMs being mood-congruent. IMs appear to be a general feature of human memory rather than just a symptom of disorders such as depression and PTSD.

REFERENCES

Andrade, J., Kavanagh, D., & Baddeley, A. (1997). Eye-movements and visual imagery: A working memory approach to the treatment of post-traumatic stress disorder. *British Journal of Clinical Psychology*, *36*, 209–223.

Baddeley, A., & Andrade, J. (2000). Working memory and the vividness of imagery. *Journal of Experimental Psychology: General*, *129*, 126–145.

Berntsen, D. (1996). Involuntary autobiographical memory. *Applied Cognitive Psychology*, *10*, 435–454.

Berntsen, D. (2001). Involuntary memories of emotional events: Do memories of traumas and extremely happy events differ? *Applied Cognitive Psychology*, *15*, 135–158.

Brewin, C. R., Christodoulides, J., & Hutchinson, G. (1996). Intrusive thoughts and intrusive memories in a nonclinical sample. *Cognition & Emotion*, *10*, 107–112.

Brewin, C. R. Dalgleish, T., & Joseph, S. (1996). A dual representation theory of post-traumatic stress disorder. *Psychological Review*, *103*, 670–686

Brewin, C. R., & Holmes, E. A. (2003). Psychological theories of posttraumatic stress disorder. *Clinical Psychology Review*, *23*, 339–376.

Brewin, C. R., Watson, M., McCarthy, S., Hyman, P., & Dayson, D. (1998). Intrusive memories and depression in cancer patients. *Behaviour Research and Therapy*, *36*, 1131–1142.

Bywaters, M., Andrade, J., & Turpin, G. (2004). Determinants of the vividness of visual imagery: The effects of delayed recall, stimulus affect and individual differences. *Memory*, *12*, 479–488.

Clements, K. (1989). The use of purpose-made electrode gels in the measurement of electrodermal activity: A correction to Grey and Smith (1984) [letter]. *Psychophysiology*, *26*, 495.

Cook, E., & Turpin, G. (1997). Differentiating orienting, startle and defence responses: The role of affect and its implications for psychopathology. In P. J. Lang, M. Balaban, & R. F. Simons (Eds.), *Attention and orienting: Sensory motivational processes* (pp. 137–164). Hillsdale, NJ: Lawrence Erlbaum Associates Inc.

Cox, B. J., Enns, M. W., Borger, S. C., & Parker, J. D. A. (1999). The nature of the depressive experience in analogue and clinically depressed samples. *Behaviour Research and Therapy*, *37*, 15–24.

Coyne, J. C. (1994). Self-reported distress: Analogue or ersatz depression? *Psychological Bulletin*, *116*, 29–45.

Eysenck, H. J., & Eysenck, S. B. G. (1969). *Personality structure and measurement*. London: Routledge & Kegan Paul.

Fridlund, A. J., & Cacioppo, J. T. (1986). Guidelines for human elecromyographic research. *Psychophysiology*, *23*, 567–589.

Grey, S. J., & Smith, B. L. (1984). A comparison between commercially available electrode gels and purpose made gel, in the measurement of electrodermal activity. *Psychophysiology*, *21*, 551–557.

Holmes, E. A., Brewin, C. R., & Hennessy, R. G. (2004). Trauma films, information processing, and developing intrusive memories. *Journal of Experimental Psychology: General*, *135*, 3–22.

Horowitz, M., Wilner, N., & Alvarez, W. (1979). Impact of Events Scale: A measure of subjective stress. *Psychosomatic Medicine*, *41*, 209–218.

Kuyken, W., & Brewin, C. R. (1994). Intrusive memories of childhood abuse during depressive episodes. *Behaviour Research and Therapy*, *32*, 525–528.

Lang, P. J., Bradley, M. M., & Cuthbert, B. N. (1998). Emotion, motivation, and anxiety: Brain mechanisms and psychophysiology. *Biological Psychiatry*, *44*, 1248–1263.

Lang, P. J., Greenwald, M. K., Bradley, M. M., & Hamm, A. O. (1993). Looking at pictures: Affective, facial, visceral, and behavioral reactions. *Psychophysiology*, *30*, 261–273.

Lang, P. J., Öhmann, A., & Vaitl, D. (1988). *The International Affective Picture System [photographic slides]*. Gainesville, FL: University of Florida, The Centre for Research in Psychophysiology.

Sheehan, P. W. (1967). A shortened form of the Betts' Questionnaire Upon Mental Imagery. *Journal of Clinical Psychology*, *23*, 386–38.

Spenceley, A., & Jerrom, W. (1997). Intrusive traumatic childhood memories in depression: A comparison between depressed, recovered, and never depressed women. *Behaviour and Cognitive Psychotherapy*, *25*, 309–318.

Spielberger, C. D., Gorsuch, R. L., Lushene, R., Vagg, P. R., & Jacobs, G. A. (1977). *State-Trait Anxiety Questionnaire*. Palo Alto, CA: Consulting Psychology Press, Inc.

Turpin, G., & Siddle, D. A. T. (1983). Effects of stimulus intensity on cardiovascular activity. *Psychophysiology*, *20*, 611–624.

Williams, J. M. G., Watts, F. N., MacLeod, C., & Mathews, A. (1997). *Cognitive psychology and emotional disorders* (2nd ed.). Chichester, UK: John Wiley & Sons Ltd

Witvliet, C. V., & Vrana, S. R. (1995). Psychophysiological responses as indices of affective dimensions. *Psychophysiology*, *32*, 436–443.

MEMORY, 2004, 12 (4), 479–488

Determinants of the vividness of visual imagery: The effects of delayed recall, stimulus affect and individual differences

Michael Bywaters, Jackie Andrade, and Graham Turpin

University of Sheffield, UK

This study investigated the influence of emotion on vividness of imagery. A total of 80 undergraduate participants saw 25 pictures from the International Affective Picture System, representing different dimensions of valence and arousal. They rated each stimulus for valence, arousal, and emotionality. Each stimulus was then presented again, and participants formed an image of it, rating the image for vividness, valence, arousal, and emotionality. During a 15-minute retention interval, participants completed several individual differences questionnaires. They then recalled each image from a verbal prompt and re-rated its quality. Slides rated as extremely valenced and highly arousing were more vividly imaged than neutral slides. Low mood was also associated with more vivid imagery. The influence of stimulus variables was greater in the immediate imagery phase; that of individual differences tended to be greater in the delayed imagery phase. Of 29 participants, 7 reported intrusive memories of highly unpleasant stimuli at 1 year follow-up.

Recent models of psychopathology have emphasised the relevance of mental imagery to the understanding and treatment of psychological disorders. They have stressed the emotional and intrusive nature of imagery and its subsequent effects on psychological wellbeing and functioning. This growth of theoretical interest in the role of imagery in psychopathology has been accompanied by empirical research into the cognitive processes underpinning imagery in certain clinical contexts. For example, Brewin and colleagues (Brewin & Saunders, 2001; Holmes, Brewin, & Hennessy, 2004) have sought evidence for separate memory systems by examining the effects of performing verbal or visuo-spatial tasks on the development of intrusive memories. In a similar vein, Andrade and colleagues (Andrade, Kavanagh, & Baddeley, 1997; Kavanagh, Freese, Andrade, & May, 2001) have tested a working memory account of a controversial therapy known as Eye Movement Desensitisation and Reprocessing.

Although research into imagery and psychopathology has gained in credibility, as shown by this special issue of *Memory*, its development has been driven by clinical theories such as that of Brewin, Dalgleish, and Joseph (1996). Most basic imagery research derives from cognitive psychology and has used studies of performance on imagery tasks to address topics such as the nature of mental representation (e.g., Kosslyn, 1994) and visuo-spatial working memory (see Logie, 1995), rather than the subjective experiences of images. Cognitive models typically do not incorporate affective processes, limiting their application to imagery in clinical domains. Studies of the cognitive basis of image vividness are limited to three research strands: (i) Cornoldi, De Beni, Cavedon, and Mazzoni (1992) studied the relationship of different stimulus characteristics to image vivid-

Correspondence should be addressed to Michael Bywaters, c/o Professor Graham Turpin, Department of Psychology, University of Sheffield, Western Bank, Sheffield S10 2TP, UK. Email: bywatm@gosh.nhs.uk

This research was conducted in partial fulfilment of a PhD by the first author at the University of Sheffield and was supported by a bequest from the Lucy Robinson Trust.

http://www.tandf.co.uk/journals/pp/09658211.html   DOI:10.1080/09658210444000160

ness, showing that image vividness is determined by image features including shape and colour, detail, context, genericity (the ease with which the image can be formed from generic information in long-term memory), and saliency; (ii) research investigating the relationship of individual differences in imagery to cognitive performance has shown a clear, but often weak, relationship between self-rated image vividness and performance on cognitive and perceptual tasks (e.g., Marks, 1973; McKelvie, 1995); (iii) Baddeley and Andrade (2000) have explored the role of memory in imagery, showing that vivid imagery requires input from modality-specific working memory systems, and also from long-term memory. A vivid visual image relies on visuo-spatial working memory resources to maintain and manipulate visual information retrieved from long-term memory. Together, these three lines of research show that whether a particular stimulus or memory can be vividly imagined depends on the specific nature of the stimulus itself, and on the availability of working memory (rather than general cognitive) resources.

An influential approach to imagery in the clinical literature is Lang's Bio-informational Theory of Imagery (Cuthbert & Lang, 1989), which aims to explain the changes that occur during imaginal and in vivo exposure treatments of phobia. Although Lang's group has advocated using imagery to study emotion, there have been no systematic investigations of the effect of emotion on the imagery experience itself. Vrana (1995) observed that pleasant images were rated as more vivid than neutral or fear images, but it was unclear whether this was due to the valence or arousal levels of the imagery. Miller, Patrick, and Levenston (2002) also found that pleasant scenes were more vivid than neutral or unpleasant scenes, but levels of pleasantness and arousal were not controlled for. Hence little is known about the effects of stimulus affect, and also of rehearsal and experience, on image vividness. We also know little about what determines whether an image becomes intrusive or distressing.

The present study obtained normative data about the relationship between the vividness of visual imagery and various stimulus and participant variables, including the affective valence and intensity of the visual stimulus cueing the imagery and individual differences in mood and imagery ability. To help link our findings with previous research, we asked participants to rate their images on rating scales used by Lang and colleagues

(arousal and valence) and by Andrade and colleagues (vividness and general emotionality). We used the International Affective Picture System (IAPS; Lang, Öhman, & Vaitl, 1988) to provide a standardised set of visual imagery cues varying in valence and arousal. This also enabled us to compare our findings with a study by Bradley, Greenwald, Petry, and Lang (1992) of the effects of valence and arousal on memory for IAPS pictures. Bradley et al. (1992) found that extremely pleasant or unpleasant stimuli, and highly arousing stimuli, are encoded better in long-term memory than more neutral stimuli; Baddeley and Andrade (2000) showed that images derived from well-encoded memories are more vivid than those from less well-encoded memories. Combining these findings, we predicted that images of highly arousing and extremely valenced stimuli would be particularly vivid.

Our study protocol comprised five phases: rating of arousal and valence of IAPS pictures; rating of images formed immediately after seeing the pictures; rating of images of verbally cued pictures after a filled retention interval; recall of IAPS pictures 1 week later; and recall after 1 year. At the 1 year follow-up, participants were also asked whether any of the images had intruded into consciousness after the experiment. The two imagery phases tested our prediction that images generated from information in working memory would be more influenced by characteristics of the original stimuli, whereas images generated from information in long-term memory would be more affected by characteristics of the individual participants. The two recall phases aimed to replicate Bradley et al.'s (1992) finding that arousing and extremely valenced pictures are more memorable than neutral pictures, and to investigate whether it is the emotionality of the stimuli that makes them memorable, or the vividness of the images that they trigger. The question about image intrusion assessed whether it was possible to induce intrusive memories from pictorial stimuli in ways similar to the use of trauma films, (e.g., Wells & Papageorgiou, 1995), and if so, to investigate the relationship between intrusions, image vividness, and the valence and arousal of the triggering stimulus.

Between the two imagery phases, participants completed measures of depression, anxiety, imagery ability, and personality. We were interested in the relationship between imagery experience and individual differences in anxiety and depression. If arousal is a determinant of image vividness, then people with high levels of state or trait anxiety may experience more vivid images than those with lower anxiety levels. If valence is a determinant of image vividness then people's tendency to retrieve particularly negative (or positive) information from memory should affect the vividness of their images. Someone who is depressed will typically recall negative information with greater ease than someone who is not depressed (e.g., Dalgleish & Watts, 1990; Matt, Vazquez & Campbell, 1992; Williams, Watts, MacLeod & Matthews, 1988), and may therefore generate particularly vivid images of negative stimuli stored in long-term memory. However, other studies (e.g., Williams & Broadbent, 1986) suggest that people with depression find it difficult to retrieve specific memories and imagery. On this basis, one would expect less vivid imagery for those who were more depressed.

METHOD

Participants

A total of 80 first-year undergraduate students (51 female, 29 male; age range 18–42) registered on a psychology module participated in the experiment in partial fulfilment of a course requirement to take part in research. They were warned that some of the stimuli were highly unpleasant before consenting to take part.

Materials

From the IAPS (Lang et al., 1988), 25 stimuli were selected with five-picture clusters chosen to sample a wide range of positions in Lang's hypothesised affective space (see Figure 1): highly pleasant and highly arousing; moderately pleasant and moderately arousing; neutral and minimally arousing; moderately unpleasant and moderately arousing; highly unpleasant and highly arousing. There were no extremely valenced but low arousal slides included in the study; there are few of these in the IAPS because valence and arousal are not completely independent. Two additional IAPS pictures were used as practice stimuli.

All stimuli and rating scales were presented individually to participants via computer. Participants indicated their responses by moving the cursor to the appropriate point of the rating scale and clicking the computer mouse. They rated

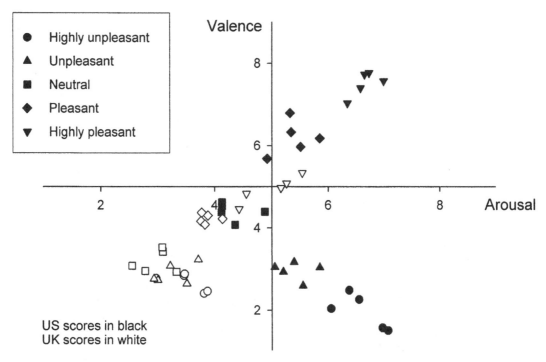

Figure 1. Distribution in affective space of the 25 IAPS slides used in this study. The filled shapes show the US normative data, according to which the stimuli were categorised for the data analysis. The unfilled shapes show the ratings made by our UK sample, for comparison.

valence and arousal on Lang's Self-Assessment Mannequin (SAM; Bradley & Lang, 1994), which comprises two separate dimensional 9-point scales made up of cartoon figures portraying valence (very pleasant to very unpleasant) and arousal (very arousing to not at all arousing). Participants rated vividness of imagery from 0 (no image at all) to 10 (image was as vivid as actual vision; Baddeley & Andrade, 2000) and emotional response from –10 (extremely negative), through 0 (neutral), to +10 (extremely positive), a measure of overall emotion used by Andrade et al. (1997; also Kavanagh et al., 2001). A pilot study verified that the verbal descriptions of slides used in the delayed imagery phase unambiguously matched one slide only.

Procedure

Participants were tested individually or in groups of up to 15 people. They completed two practice sessions. Instructions for the picture rating and immediate imagery phases were presented on screen for 40 seconds before the experimental session began. For the *picture rating* phase, participants viewed and rated each of the 25 IAPS pictures. On each trial, a screen prepared the participants for the following IAPS picture and reminded them to view the image for the entire time that it was presented. This instruction was presented for 2 seconds, followed by an IAPS picture for 6 seconds. Computerised rating screens then appeared for 8 seconds each, the first requesting a rating of emotional response to the picture and the second asking for SAM ratings of the picture's valence and arousal (position of valence/arousal scale at top/bottom of screen was counterbalanced).

In the *immediate imagery* phase, participants viewed the IAPS pictures again and rated their images of them. This phase was identical to the rating phase, except that after viewing each picture participants closed their eyes and tried to image it as vividly as they could. After 6 seconds of imaging, a tone cued participants to open their eyes. Participants then rated the vividness of their image, followed by the emotional impact, valence, and arousal of the image. Vividness was always rated first to gain as accurate a measure as possible of vividness of imagery (see Cornoldi et al., 1992). Rating scales remained on screen for 8 seconds.

Participants then completed the Beck Depression Inventory (BDI; Beck, Ward, Mendelson,

Mock, & Erbaugh, 1961), a shortened version of the Eysenck Personality Questionnaire (EPQ; Eysenck & Eysenck, 1969), the Spielberger State-Trait Anxiety Inventory (STAI; Spielberger, Gorsuch, Lushene, Vagg, & Jacobs, 1977), and the shortened version of the Betts' Questionnaire upon Mental Imagery (QMI; Sheehan, 1967). This phase lasted approximately 15 minutes. Participants were not told at this time about the subsequent delayed imagery phase.

The *delayed imagery* phase was identical to the immediate imagery phase, except that participants viewed a verbal description of the pictures rather than the pictures themselves. Participants were instructed: "From the description given below, please decide which slide this best describes that you have seen previously in this experiment. When the screen goes blank, please close your eyes and try to imagine the slide, until you hear the tone." Participants imaged the slide for 6 seconds and then rated the image on vividness and overall emotional response (first screen), and arousal and valence (second screen), as before. Stimuli were presented in a different random order for each phase of the experiment and for each participant. Participants were debriefed and thanked for their participation.

One week later, participants were contacted by email and asked to respond with a description of all of the slides that they could remember. They were also emailed approximately 1 year after completing the experiment and again asked to recall as many of the slides as they could, stating whether any of the images seen during the experiment had intruded as intrusive memories, defined as "memories of a specific event or incident that has happened to you sometime previously. They can be pleasant (positive) or unpleasant (negative) memories that interrupt day to day activity and may be difficult to control" (Brewin, Christodoulides, & Hutchinson, 1996, p. 108).

Data quantification and analysis

Participants occasionally failed to make a rating within the 15 seconds allowed. They were excluded from the analysis if they had missing data from one or more of the averaged valence categories. Five participants' data were thus excluded, leaving a final sample size of 75.

As expected from the selection of slides, the relationship between valence ratings and vividness was non-linear (i.e., both extremely pleasant and extremely unpleasant images were rated as very vivid as compared to more neutral images), thus the raw scores could not be used in any correlational analysis between valence and vividness. The "overall emotion" and valence scores showed two linear patterns either side of zero (the central point on the scale). Scores on these scales were therefore recoded by calculating the distance from the score to the mid-point of the scale. Thus negative (unpleasant) ratings became positive "valence magnitude" and "strength of emotion" scores (Andrade et al., 1997). This transformation revealed a linear relationship between valence and vividness, and overall emotion and vividness. The transformed scores are used throughout the correlational analyses.

Several approaches were adopted towards the data analysis: ANOVA was employed to assess the effects of stimulus attributes on imagery ratings in each phase of the study. For each participant, mean scores were calculated for each of the five IAPS picture categories for each rating scale. Thus each participant had one vividness score for highly pleasant stimuli/images, one for pleasant, and so on. Greenhouse-Geisser Epsilon correction was used as a conservative measure of significance level, and all p values reported are using this correction. We checked that the valence/arousal categories (as defined by the IAPS ratings) were similar when rated by UK students, despite differences in rating behaviour between the UK and US samples.

We used correlations to examine the consistency of ratings across the experimental period, and to test relationships between participants' picture ratings (rather than normative IAPS categorisations) and subsequent imagery ratings. A mean score for each IAPS picture was obtained for each rating scale by taking the mean of all participants' scores for that picture and that scale. Ratings for the immediate and delayed imagery trials for each picture were likewise averaged across participants. Note that a low score on the arousal scale relates to a highly arousing slide (i.e., the SAM icon indicating highest arousal was scored as 1, and the lowest arousal as 9). For the other scales, a high score equates to a high rating.

Individual differences were explored with correlations and multiple regressions, using data processed as for the main ANOVAs. The follow up recall data were analysed using one-way ANOVA.

RESULTS

IAPS ratings

A preliminary analysis showed that the UK students generally rated the slides as less arousing and less strongly pleasant/unpleasant than did the US sample. The overall ranking of the slides was roughly similar, with general agreement on what was pleasant and what was not (further details available from the first author).

Effects of picture category on valence, arousal, overall emotion, and vividness. Participants' averaged ratings on the valence, arousal, and overall emotion scales were subjected to 5 (picture category) × 3 (experimental period) repeated measures ANOVAs. The results of these analyses are reported briefly because they essentially show that we had, as intended, selected distinct categories of IAPS pictures. A significance level of 5% is assumed. The valence ratings showed a highly significant effect of category and a significant interaction between category and period. This interaction was due to the range of scores being slightly restricted for the imagery phases of the experiment when compared with the slide-rating phase. The analysis of the overall emotion ratings gave a similar pattern of results. The arousal ratings showed significant main effects of category and period, and a significant interaction. The highly pleasant and highly unpleasant slides were rated as more arousing than the less extremely valenced slides. In contrast to the valence ratings, the difference in arousal ratings across categories became less pronounced from the picture-rating phase to the delayed imagery phase.

Table 1 shows the vividness of imagery scores for the immediate and delayed imagery periods. These scores were subjected to a 5 × 2 ANOVA with picture category and period (immediate or delayed) as within-subjects factors. The effect of picture category was highly significant, $F(4, 296) = 27.86$, $p < .001$. Post hoc comparisons revealed that all the categories differed significantly from each other ($p < .05$), except the highly pleasant and unpleasant categories, and the highly unpleasant and pleasant categories (n.s.). The highly pleasant pictures were imaged most vividly, followed by unpleasant, highly unpleasant, and pleasant pictures. Images of neutral pictures were rated least vivid. There was no effect of imagery period on vividness, $F(1, 74) = 2.51$, $p = .097$, and no interaction between period and category, $F(4, 296) = 1.88$, $p = .155$.

TABLE 1
Vividness ratings

Picture category	Immediate ratings	Delayed ratings
Highly pleasant	6.95 (1.61)	6.51 (1.72)
Pleasant	5.84 (1.69)	5.85 (1.75)
Neutral	5.61 (1.74)	5.55 (1.85)
Unpleasant	6.24 (1.65)	6.07 (1.86)
Highly unpleasant	6.18 (1.71)	5.93 (1.92)

Mean vividness of imagery ratings for the five categories of IAPS pictures, immediately after viewing the picture and after a filled retention interval (± standard deviations).

Correlational analysis

Correlations between picture ratings and vividness of imagery. We used two-tailed correlations to test the prediction that pictures that had been rated as extremely valenced and highly arousing would be imaged more vividly than those rated as more neutral. Supporting this prediction, picture valence ratings were significantly correlated with vividness at the immediate, $r(23) = .67, p < .001$, and delayed, $r(23) = .54, p < .01$, imagery phases, with the more emotionally charged slides leading to more vivid images. Arousal ratings for the pictures were similarly correlated with image vividness, $r(23) = .59, p < .01$ for immediate imagery and $r(23) = .54, p < .01$ for delayed imagery. Images of more arousing slides were rated as more vivid than those of less arousing slides. "Overall emotion" ratings for pictures also significantly correlated with image vividness, both at the immediate and delayed imagery phases, $r(23) = .78, p < .001$, and $r(23) = .62, p < .001$ respectively.

For both valence and overall emotion, the correlation with image vividness was stronger for the immediate imagery period than for the delayed imagery period, $r(23) = .45, p < .05$ and $r(23) = .49, p < .01$ respectively. This suggests that the influence of the initial stimulus characteristics on vividness diminishes as the image becomes more dependent on long-term memory. The correlations between arousal and vividness were slightly but not significantly higher for the immediate imagery period than for the delayed period.

Correlations between vividness and emotionality of images. For both the immediate and the delayed imagery periods, images rated as highly arousing were very vivid, $r(23) = -.73, p < .001$, and $r(23) = -.63, p < .001$ respectively. Images rated as extremely valenced were also very vivid for the immediate and for the delayed imagery periods $r(23) = .81, p < .001$, and $r(23) = .65, p < .001$ respectively. There were strong correlations between the ratings of the overall emotion of images and image vividness, for immediate and delayed imagery, $r(23) = .80, p < .001$, and $r(23) = .67, p < .001$ respectively.

Correlations of "overall emotion" ratings with valence and arousal ratings of slides and images. Ratings of "overall emotion" on the scale used by Andrade et al. (1997) correlated strongly with ratings of the slides on Lang's scales of valence, $r(23) = .98, p < .001$, and arousal, $r(23) = -.68, p < .001$. This was also true for immediate imagery, $r(23) = .99, p < .001$ for valence and $r(23) = -.84, p < .001$ for arousal. For delayed imagery, overall emotion correlated with arousal but not valence, $r(23) = -.89, p < .001$, $r(23) = .29, p = .15$. respectively.

Contribution of individual differences to vividness of imagery

Multiple regressions assessed the contribution of individual differences to the vividness of imagery. Only four analyses were conducted, to examine the most extreme cases (immediate and delayed imagery of highly pleasant and unpleasant pictures) while minimising the chance of type I errors. The dependent variable in each case was the mean vividness for each picture category, as calculated for the ANOVAs above. The independent variables were picture valence rating, BDI score, STAI score (state anxiety score), and imagery ability score (the sum of the visual imagery scores from the QMI). There was an extremely high correlation between valence and arousal scores for each of the valence groups, so arousal was excluded from the analysis to avoid problems of multicolinearity. Valence was used rather than arousal in the regressions as there was a higher correlation between valence and vividness than between arousal and vividness.

For immediate imagery of the highly pleasant pictures, the regression was significant, $F(4, 70) = 4.20, p < .01$, with an adjusted r^2 value of .14. Beta weights showed that BDI score and valence made significant individual contributions to variance ($p < .01$), with low mood and extreme valence slides leading to more vivid images. Similar results were obtained for delayed, highly pleasant imagery.

The regression was highly significant, $F(4, 70) = 5.57$, $p < .001$, with an adjusted r^2 value of .20. Valence ($p < .01$) and BDI score ($p < .05$) made significant individual contributions to variance, again with extreme valence and low mood leading to increased vividness.

For immediate imagery of the highly unpleasant slides, the regression was significant, $F(4, 70) = 3.69$, $p < .01$; adjusted $r^2 = .13$, and beta weights showed that valence ($p < .05$) and BDI score ($p = .05$) made significant individual contributions to variance. The regression was also highly significant for delayed imagery of the highly unpleasant slides, $F(4, 70) = 5.70$, $p < .001$; adjusted $r^2 = .20$. Beta weights showed that the BDI score, STAI score, and imagery ability score all made significant individual contributions to vividness ($p < .05$, $p < .01$, and $p < .05$ respectively). Low mood, high imagery ability, and high state anxiety led to more vivid imagery. Valence did not contribute significantly to vividness in this regression.

Although these regressions are all significant, they have relatively low r^2 values. The reason for this is the very restricted range of scores in the regression, due to the scores having already been sorted by their valence category. Given this fact, it seems interesting that we have obtained any significant individual contributions at all from the independent variables. Valence contributed significantly to vividness in three of the four regressions and BDI score contributed significantly in all four regressions. Inspection of the beta weights suggests that the contribution of BDI is largest for the delayed imagery, highly unpleasant condition. This is concordant with our hypotheses that the effect of individual differences will be greater for images based on information stored in long-term memory, and that people with low mood will generate particularly vivid images of negative stimuli because of mood-congruency effects in retrieval from long-term memory.

Analysis of the individual differences revealed that there was a strong correlation between depression levels and levels of state anxiety, $r(73) = .64$, $p < .001$. There were also strong correlations between the neuroticism score from the EPQ and depression level, $r(73) = .57$, $p < .001$, and between neuroticism and anxiety level, $r(73) = .56$, $p < .001$. There was no correlation between imagery ability and depression, anxiety, or neuroticism score, $r(73) = .09$, .05, and .08 respectively.

Recall at 1 week and 1 year

A total of 37 participants, just under half the sample, responded to the email prompting recall at 1 week after participation. The slides recalled by each participant were categorised according to their IAPS valence and arousal ratings. The analysis was conducted on the proportion of slides recalled in each valence category by each person (see Bradley et al., 1992). Repeated measures ANOVA showed a highly significant effect of valence on recall, $F(4, 144) = 17.35$, $p < .001$. Tukey's HSD post-hoc analyses revealed poorer recall from the neutral category than the other categories apart from the unpleasant category, and better recall of highly pleasant than pleasant and highly unpleasant than unpleasant slides. There was a significant effect of arousal category, $F(2, 72) = 138.78$, $p < .001$, with Tukey's HSD analyses showing significant differences between all the categories ($p < .001$ for all differences). More arousing slides were more likely to be recalled than less arousing slides (Table 2).

A total of 29 participants responded to the 1 year follow-up asking about recall and intrusions. Repeated measures ANOVA again showed a significant effect of valence category on the proportion of slides recalled, $F(4, 26) = 15.77$, $p < .001$. Tukey's HSD analyses revealed that highly unpleasant slides were recalled significantly better than any other category, with no significant differences between the other categories (see Table 2). Repeated measures ANOVA also showed a significant effect of arousal, $F(2, 72) = 138.78$, $p < .001$. Tukey's HSD post-hoc analyses revealed

TABLE 2
Arousal and valence

Arousal category	Valence category	One week (n = 37)	One year (n = 29)
High arousal	Highly pleasant	0.241 (0.065)	0.221 (0.262)
	Highly unpleasant	0.270 (0.074)	0.535 (0.332)
Medium arousal	Pleasant	0.193 (0.070)	0.139 (0.239)
	Unpleasant	0.168 (0.085)	0.077 (0.180)
Low arousal	Neutral	0.128 (0.073)	0.028 (0.083)

Mean proportion of slides recalled by *valence* and *arousal* category, and retention interval (± standard deviation).

significant differences between all the arousal categories.

A total of 7 (24%) of the 29 respondents reported that at least one of the slides had intruded since participating in the experiment. All the intrusions were from slides in the highly unpleasant valence category as rated in the IAPS.

DISCUSSION

Participants viewed a range of affective stimuli from the IAPS and rated them for arousal, valence, and emotionality. They then formed mental images of these stimuli and rated the images for arousal, valence, emotionality, and vividness, once immediately after viewing the slides and once cued by a textual prompt after a delay. We observed effects of stimulus characteristics and individual differences on image vividness, as discussed below. The affective properties of the slides influenced recall at 1 week and 1 year follow-up. Some participants at 1 year follow-up reported intrusive visual images of the highly unpleasant stimuli.

The contribution of stimulus affect to image vividness

We believe our study to be the first systematic investigation of the relationship between emotional valence and image vividness. The results show a strong contribution of valence to vividness, with highly pleasant and highly unpleasant images being more vivid than neutral images. There were significant effects of picture category on vividness of images of the pictures, and strong correlations between valence (of pictures and images) and vividness. There were also strong correlations between arousal and vividness and between overall emotionality and vividness.

The contribution of valence, and of overall emotion, to imagery vividness might most parsimoniously be explained in terms of arousal, because the extremely valenced stimuli are also highly arousing. Bradley et al. (1992) found that, when arousal was taken into account, valence made no additional contribution to recall of IAPS slides after 1 week (although highly unpleasant slides were recalled better after 1 year). Thompson (1985) reported a similar finding when looking at memory for naturally occurring events. Bradley et al. (1992) suggested that arousing stimuli were easier to recall because they underwent greater elaboration at encoding. Given Baddeley and Andrade's (2000) hypothesis that vividness of imagery reflects ease of retrieval of relevant sensory information from memory, this greater elaboration and subsequent good recall may also account for the greater vividness of images of arousing stimuli.

The contribution of individual differences to image vividness

We predicted that, if valence were an important determinant of image vividness, then participants' mood would also contribute to vividness such that low mood would facilitate vivid imagery of unpleasant stimuli and high mood would facilitate imagery of pleasant stimuli. BDI scores did indeed correlate with image vividness but, contrary to our prediction, people with low mood rated their pleasant, as well as unpleasant, images as more vivid than did those with high mood, even when taking into account overall imagery ability. This finding is partially supported by our study of autobiographical memory that found depressed mood participants had more vivid imagery for both pleasant and unpleasant intrusive memories, and unpleasant non-intrusive memories (Bywaters, Andrade, & Turpin, 2004 this issue). However that study did show some evidence of mood congruency in vividness ratings, with non-depressed mood participants having more vivid imagery for pleasant non-intrusive memories.

Although there are problems in generalising these results to depressed populations, we note that 30 of our 75 participants had BDI scores of 9 or above. Cox, Enns, Borger, and Parker (1999) compared analogue and clinical samples based on the phenomenology of their depressive experience, using a cut-off of 9 on the BDI. They concluded that the differences found between their samples were of a quantitative rather than qualitative nature: their analysis indicated that the symptom structure of the analogue and clinical samples was very similar, differing only in severity.

Determinants of image vividness: Change over time

We have identified two influences on imagery vividness: the affective properties of the stimulus and the mood of the individual. Further research is needed to determine whether the effects of the mood of the participant can be separated from the emotion inherent in the stimulus itself. For example, one could use mood induction techniques or induce arousal through exercise prior to imagery, or manipulate valence of a stimulus (e.g., a football match) by changing its interpretation (supporters of the winners versus those of the losers).

Our findings suggest that another way of separating the influences of stimulus and participant characteristics on imagery is through the passage of time. The correlations between valence and vividness, and overall emotion and vividness, were significantly stronger at the immediate imagery phase than at the delayed imagery phase. Stimulus characteristics appear to be particularly important for immediate imagery, based predominantly on information held in working memory. As time passes, and imagery relies more on long-term memory, the influence of stimulus characteristics on vividness appears to wane and that of individual differences grows. This can be seen in the multiple regression data, with the individual differences all contributing significantly for the highly unpleasant delayed imagery, whereas valence did not.

We suggest that the momentary increase in arousal induced by viewing a highly pleasant or unpleasant stimulus may particularly enhance storage of that stimulus in working memory, enabling veridical features of the stimulus to be incorporated into the image when imagery occurs immediately after viewing the stimulus. With a delay between viewing and imaging the stimulus, there is still better retrieval of the original arousing images than more neutral ones due to the greater elaboration, but some memory for precise details of these stimuli will be lost and therefore imagery becomes more dependent on retrieval of generic information from long-term memory. This retrieval is sensitive to individual differences (although we expected, but did not find, mood-congruent effects on delayed imagery).

Recall data

Recall at 1 week follow-up replicated Bradley et al.'s (1992) finding, showing that stimulus affect mediates delayed recall. Highly pleasant and unpleasant stimuli were more likely to be recalled than neutral stimuli. At the 1 year follow-up there was an effect of valence such that highly unpleasant slides were recalled better than the other stimuli. This is particularly interesting given that

these slides were rated as less extremely valenced than the highly pleasant slides.

Highly arousing traumatic events are often the basis for intrusive negative memories, and these memories might in turn lead to further decreases in mood. Elevated anxiety and depression are associated with many social and occupational consequences of serious physical trauma (Mason, Wardrope, Turpin, & Rowlands, 2002a, 2002b). If negative mood is related to increased imagery vividness, as the present findings suggest (see also Bywaters et al., 2004 this issue), this could lead to an increase in vivid negative and intrusive imagery, and further worsening of mood in a vicious circle serving the maintenance of depression following traumatic events. There is evidence that intrusive images abate when people recover from depressive episodes, but levels of avoidance remain high (Spenceley & Jerrom, 1997). Intrusive memories may remain a risk factor for relapse into depression. If individuals are vulnerable to vivid intrusions, decreases in mood or increases in arousal levels may trigger further intrusive memories, which may in turn lead to further depressive episodes. We feel the relationship between vivid imagery, intrusive memories, and mood and arousal warrants further investigation.

In conclusion, the findings suggest that vividness of imagery is influenced by the affective properties of the triggering stimulus and by the mood state of the individual performing the imagining. More arousing and highly valenced stimuli were imaged more vividly than neutral stimuli, and depressed mood was associated with more vivid imagery of both positive and negative materials. The relative contributions of these stimulus variables and individual differences changed over time, a finding that we interpret as reflecting changes in the cognitive processes underlying imagery. When participants image a stimulus that has just been presented, their image is based largely on information held in working memory (Baddeley & Andrade, 2000) and is more susceptible to the emotional qualities of the stimulus. When there is a longer delay between perceiving the stimulus and forming an image of it, the image is based on information held in long-term memory and is more susceptible to the emotional status of the participant, which influences accessibility of emotive information from LTM. Theories of imagery should take account of the nature of the imagery stimulus, the emotional status of the person performing the imagery, and the type of memory from which the image is derived.

REFERENCES

Andrade, J., Kavanagh, D., & Baddeley, A. (1997). Eye-movements and visual imagery: A working memory approach to the treatment of post-traumatic stress disorder. *British Journal of Clinical Psychology, 36,* 209–223.

Baddeley, A., & Andrade, J. (2000). Working memory and the vividness of imagery. *Journal of Experimental Psychology: General, 129,* 126–145.

Beck, A. T., Ward, C. H., Mendelson, M., Mock, J., & Erbaugh, J. (1961). An inventory for measuring depression. *Archives of General Psychiatry, 4,* 561–571.

Bradley, M. M., Greenwald, M. K., Petry, M. C., & Lang, P. J. (1992). Remembering pictures: Pleasure and arousal in memory. *Journal of Experimental Psychology: Learning, Memory and Cognition, 18,* 379–390.

Bradley, M. M., & Lang, P. J. (1994). Measuring emotion: The self-assessment manikin and the semantic differential. *Journal of Behaviour and Experimental Psychiatry, 25,* 49–59.

Brewin, C. R., Christodoulides, J., & Hutchinson, G. (1996). Intrusive thoughts and memories in a non-clinical sample. *Cognition and Emotion, 10,* 107–112.

Brewin, C. R., Dalgleish, T., & Joseph, S. (1996). A dual representation theory of posttraumatic stress disorder. *Psychological Review, 103,* 1–17.

Brewin, C. R., & Saunders, J. (2001). The effect of dissociation at encoding on intrusive memories for a stressful film. *British Journal of Medical Psychology, 74,* 467–472.

Bywaters, M. J., Andrade, J., & Turpin, G. (2004). Intrusive and non-intrusive memories in a non-clinical sample: The effects of mood and affect on imagery vividness. *Memory, 12,* 467–478.

Cornoldi, C., De Beni, R., Cavedon, A., & Mazzoni, G. (1992). How can a vivid image be described? Characteristics influencing vividness judgments and the relationship between vividness and memory. *Journal of Mental Imagery, 16,* 89–108.

Cox, B. J., Enns, M. W., Borger, S. C., & Parker, J. D. A. (1999). The nature of the depressive experience in analogue and clinically depressed samples. *Behaviour Research and Therapy, 37,* 15–24.

Cuthbert, B. N., & Lang, P.J. (1989). Imagery, memory, and emotion: A psychophysiological analysis of clinical anxiety. In G. Turpin (Ed.), *Handbook of clinical psychophysiology* (pp. 105–134). Chichester, UK: Wiley.

Dalgleish, T., & Watts, F. N. (1990). Biases of attention and memory in disorders of anxiety and depression. *Clinical Psychology Review, 10,* 589–604.

Eysenck, H. J., & Eysenck, S. B. G. (1969). *Personality structure and measurement.* London: Routledge & Kegan Paul.

Holmes, E., Brewin, C. R., & Hennessy, R. D. (2004). Trauma films, information processing and intrusive memory development. *Journal of Experimental Psychology: General, 135,* 3–22.

Kavanagh, G. J., Freese, S., Andrade, J., & May, J. (2001). Effects of visuospatial tasks on desensitisation to emotive memories. *British Journal of Clinical Psychology, 40,* 267–280.

Kosslyn, S. M. (1994) *Image and brain: The resolution of the imagery debate.* Cambridge, MA: MIT Press.

Lang, P. J., Öhmann, A., & Vaitl, D. (1988). *The International Affective Picture System [photographic slides].* Gainesville, FL: University of Florida, The Centre for Research in Psychophysiology.

Logie, R. H. (1995). *Visuo-spatial working memory.* Hove, UK: Lawrence Erlbaum Associates Ltd.

Marks, D. F. (1973). Visual imagery differences in the recall of pictures. *British Journal of Psychology, 64,* 17–24.

Mason, S., Wardrope, J., Turpin, G., & Rowlands, A. (2002a). Outcomes following injury: A comparison of workplace and non-workplace injury. *The Journal of Trauma, 53,* 98–103.

Mason, S., Wardrope, J., Turpin, G., & Rowlands, A. (2002b). The psychological burden of injury: An eighteen month prospective cohort study. *Emergency Medicine Journal, 19,* 400–404.

Matt, G. E., Vazquez, C., & Campbell, W. K. (1992). Mood congruent recall of affectively toned stimuli: A meta-analytic review. *Clinical Psychology Review, 12,* 227–255.

McKelvie, S. J. (1995). The VVIQ as a psychometric test of individual differences in visual imagery vividness: A critical quantitative review and plea for direction. *Journal of Mental Imagery, 19,* 1–106.

Merckelbach, H., Hogervorst, E., Kampman, M. C., & De Jong, A. (1994). Effects of eye movement desensitisation on emotional processing in normal subjects. *Behavioural and Cognitive Psychotherapy, 22,* 331–335.

Miller, M. W., Patrick, C. J., & Levenston, G. K. (2002). Affective imagery and the startle response: Probing mechanisms of modulation during pleasant scenes, personal experiences, and discrete negative emotions. *Psychophysiology, 39,* 519–529.

Sheehan, P. W. (1967). A shortened form of the Betts' Questionnaire Upon Mental Imagery. *Journal of Clinical Psychology, 23,* 386–389.

Spenceley, A., & Jerrom, W. (1997). Intrusive traumatic childhood memories in depression: A comparison between depressed, recovered, and never depressed women. *Behavioural and Cognitive Psychotherapy, 25,* 309–318.

Spielberger, C. D., Gorsuch, R. L., Lushene, R., Vagg, P. R., & Jacobs, G. A. (1977). *Stait-Trait Anxiety Questionnaire.* Palo Alto, CA: Consulting Psychology Press, Inc.

Thompson, C. P. (1985). Memory for unique personal events: Effects of pleasantness. *Motivation and Emotion, 9,* 277–289.

Vrana, S. R. (1995). Emotional modulation of skin conductance and eye-blink responses to a startle probe. *Psychophysiology, 32,* 351–357.

Wells, A., & Papageorgiou, C. (1995). Worry and the incubation of intrusive images following stress. *Behaviour Research and Therapy, 33,* 579–583.

Williams, J. M. G., & Broadbent, K. (1986). Autobiographical memory in suicide attempters. *Journal of Abnormal Psychology, 95,* 144–149.

Williams, J. M. G., Watts, F. N., MacLeod, C., & Matthews, A. (1988). *Cognitive psychology and emotional disorders.* Chichester, UK: Wiley.

MEMORY, 2004, *12* (4), 489–495

Memory perspective and self-concept in social anxiety: An exploratory study

Lusia Stopa and Tess Bryant

University of Southampton, UK

The mental representation of self and observer perspective images are important maintaining factors in cognitive models of social phobia (Clark & Wells, 1995; Rapee & Heimberg, 1997). This study investigates Libby and Eibach's (2002) hypothesis that the observer perspective is used to recall memories that are incongruent with current self-concept. A total of 60 participants (divided into high and low social anxiety groups) completed a questionnaire in which they described current self-concept, recalled four memories of social occasions (two congruent, two incongruent), and rated memory age and vividness. Congruence was defined as memories that "fit" with current self-descriptions. A qualitative analysis of self-concept showed that both groups used a similar range of themes. High socially anxious participants recalled more observer perspective memories in the second incongruent memory. Congruence did not influence vividness, but public self-consciousness did. The implications of the results are discussed and suggestions made for future research.

Cognitive models of social phobia (Clark & Wells, 1995; Rapee & Heimberg, 1997) propose that self-focused attention and the construction of a mental representation of self maintain social anxiety. Clark and Wells argue that socially phobic individuals shift to detailed observation and monitoring of the self when faced with the prospect of negative evaluation, and generate a negative impression of how they appear to others, constructed from their own thoughts, feelings, and internal sensations. This impression can occur in the form of a visual image that is seen from an external, or "observer" perspective. Rapee and Heimberg also suggest that individuals develop a mental representation of the self in social situations.

Recent evidence demonstrates that socially phobic individuals remember social situations more often from an observer perspective than from a field perspective (seeing the image from behind your own eyes) compared to non-anxious individuals (Coles, Turk, Heimberg, & Fresco, 2001; Hackmann, Surawy, & Clark, 1998; Wells, Clark, & Ahmad, 1998; Wells & Papageorgiou, 1999). External focus during exposure reduced use of the observer perspective (Wells & Papageorgiou, 1998), and viewing videotapes of speeches using the observer perspective improved self-ratings of performance in high, but not low, socially anxious individuals (Spurr & Stopa, 2003).

Negative images also play an important maintaining role in social anxiety. Hackmann, Clark, and McManus (2000) interviewed 22 patients with social phobia; the participants all reported spontaneously recurring negative images. Hirsch, Clark, Mathews, and Williams (2003) showed that socially phobic patients rated anxiety higher, performance worse, and believed their anxiety was more visible if they held a negative image in mind during a conversation with a stranger compared to a less negative control image.

Correspondence should be sent to Dr Lusia Stopa, Department of Psychology, University of Southampton, Highfield, Southampton SO17 1BJ, UK. Email: L.Stopa@soton.ac.uk

The research reported in this paper was supported by a Faculty of Social Science Research Support Grant (Reference: D10 0434) from the University of Southampton.

http://www.tandf.co.uk/journals/pp/09658211.html   DOI:10.1080/09658210444000098

Both cognitive models (Clark & Wells, 1995; Rapee & Heimberg, 1997) agree that the mental representation of self is constructed from multiple inputs. Clark (2001) suggests three types of input: information derived from anxiety symptoms, spontaneously occurring images, and a "felt sense" (Clark, 2001, p. 408). Rapee and Heimberg (1997) propose that self-representations draw on images stored in long-term memory that are modified on-line in response to proprioceptive and somatic information, and feedback from other people. Empirical evidence to support these claims is limited. Although Hackmann et al.'s (2000) study indicated that self-representations may be influenced by stored images, Wells and Papageorgiou (2001) failed to support their prediction that information about bodily state, delivered through a false pulse-rate feedback manipulation, would affect perspective taking in patients with generalised social phobia.

Neither model specifies the factors that determine memory perspective. Early work by Nigro and Neisser (1983) is useful in this respect. Nigro and Neisser demonstrated that older memories, instructions to focus on the objective circumstances of the memory, and memories with a high degree of emotional self-awareness are more likely to be remembered from an observer perspective. More recent memories and a focus on feelings rather than on objective circumstances increase use of the field perspective. The effects of switching perspective are asymmetrical: shifting from field to observer reduced affect, whereas switching from observer to field did not (Robinson & Swanson, 1993).

The increased frequency of observer perspective memories in social phobia might be due to memory age. Hackmann et al. (2000) showed that many memories dated back to the age of onset of the disorder. However, self-consciousness and self-focused attention also increase use of the observer perspective (Libby & Eibach, 2002), so choice of perspective is unlikely to be attributable to a single factor. Libby and Eibach suggested that decisions about perspective are made on-line and depend on the perception of a discrepancy between the remembered behaviours and current self-schemas. They argued that individuals use the observer perspective when remembering actions that are incongruent with their current view of self. The relationship between autobiographical memory and self-concept is a key feature of Conway's work, and Conway and Pleydell-Pearce (2000) stress the fundamental importance of autobiographical memory to the individual's sense of self, although they do not discuss the role of perspective.

Libby and Eibach (2002) conducted a series of experiments that included asking individuals to remember situations that were discrepant with current self-view, for example, remembering aspects of the self that had changed most or least since high school, and predicting future behaviours (e.g., overeating) after remembering similar incidents in the past. Participants used the observer perspective more often when imaging events/behaviours that conflicted with current self-view and were more optimistic about not overeating if they remembered previous instances of overeating from an observer perspective. Libby and Eibach concluded that the "on-line perception of inconsistency causes the third-person memory perspective" (p. 176). They argued that the past self is seen as another person, and this is translated literally into the visual perspective of another person.

Can these suggestions help to explain the increased frequency of the observer perspective in social phobia? Clark and Wells (1995) argue that socially phobic individuals, unlike depressed individuals, have unstable self-schemas and only see themselves negatively when social anxiety activates a negative self-view. At other times the individual has a relatively positive or adaptive view of self. Interview studies of the observer perspective may not have activated negative self-schemas, and therefore memories of high anxious social situations could have been perceived as incongruent. This hypothesis could be tested by asking participants to remember events before and after a social threat activation task. Alternatively, incongruence may occur because remembered actions conflict with an idealised and unrealistic view of the self.

The current study was an exploratory investigation of whether congruence with current self-concept influenced the use of perspective in high and low socially anxious individuals. Participants generated descriptions of self-concept and then recalled four memories—two congruent and two incongruent. We predicted that the high socially anxious group would use the observer perspective more overall, but that both groups would use the observer perspective more in the incongruent than in the congruent condition. The study also investigated the themes selected to describe self-concept using a qualitative analysis, examined whether vividness differed in congruent and incongruent memories, and looked at the impact of self-consciousness on memory vividness.

METHOD

Participants

A total of 60 undergraduate and postgraduate students at the University of Southampton completed the experiment for course credits or payment of £5.00. The sample was divided into high (5 men and 25 women) and low (4 men and 26 women) social anxiety groups on the basis of a median split (MD = 15.5) on the Fear of Negative Evaluation Scale (FNES: Watson & Friend, 1969). The mean FNES scores were 22.33 (SD = 4.27) and 8.6 (SD = 3.30) respectively.

Measures and procedure

Self-concept and memory questionnaire. The memory questionnaire comprised three sections. In part 1, participants read a list of 26 positive and negative self-descriptors, circled words that described them, and then wrote a description of themselves. In part 2, participants recalled two congruent and two incongruent memories (counterbalanced). Congruent memories were those that "fit well with the description that you have just given of yourself", whereas incongruent memories were those where "you either felt or behaved very differently from the way you have just described". In part 3, participants rated perspective (observer, field, or neither), recorded memory age, and rated vividness on a 0 (not at all vivid) to 5 (extremely vivid) scale. Questionnaires were completed individually and returned to the experimenter. The questionnaire is available from the authors.

Fear of Negative Evaluation Scale (FNES). The FNES is a 30-item true–false inventory that measures fear of negative evaluation by others. It has good internal consistency, test–retest reliability, and discriminant validity (Watson & Friend, 1969). Participants with high FNES scores perform similarly on cognitive measures to patients with social phobia and therefore provide a reasonable analogue to social phobia (Stopa & Clark, 2001).

Self-Consciousness Scale-Revised (SCS-R). The SCS-R is a 22-item self-report scale that measures public and private self-consciousness and social anxiety (Scheier & Carver, 1985). Private self-consciousness describes awareness of inner thoughts, feelings, and attitudes, whereas public self-consciousness describes awareness of the publicly observable aspects of self. Items are rated on a 0 (extremely uncharacteristic) to 4 (extremely characteristic) scale. The three sub-scales have good levels of internal consistency and reasonable levels of test–retest reliability.

RESULTS

Participant characteristics

A total of 60 participants completed the questionnaire packs. The high socially anxious group scored significantly higher than the low socially anxious group on public self-consciousness (high anxious M = 15.6, SD = 3.5, low anxious M = 9.1, SD = 4.3; t = 6.41, $p < .001$, d = 1.66) and private self-consciousness (high anxious M = 17.9, SD = 4.4, low anxious M = 13.1, SD = 4.9; t = 4.01, $p < .001$, d = 1.03) on the SCS-R; and on the social anxiety sub-scale of the SCS-R (high anxious M = 11.0, SD = 3.8, low anxious M = 7.7, SD = 3.8; t = 3.39, $p < .001$, d = 0.87).

Self-concept descriptions

A thematic analysis (Joffe & Yardley, 2004) of the participants' self-descriptions produced 10 categories. *Participation* referred to both active (looking for things in common or finding out new things from people) and passive (being there but not taking an active role) involvement in activities. "*True self*" referred to differences between a "true" self and what other people may see, and to acting in opposition to the way one felt. *Enjoyment* referred to pleasure and degree of effort in social situations. *Confident/shy* referred to being or not being confident or shy. *Talkative/lively/outgoing* included references to any of these qualities. *Stability* referred to the consistency of the self across situations, for example, the idea that you are different type of person according to the situation. "Stable" was coded for single descriptions of the self; "unstable" for more than one description. *Factors affecting descriptions of self* referred to situational and interpersonal factors that affected feelings or behaviour in social situations. *Importance of other people's opinions* described being positively or negatively evaluated by others. *Acceptance* described acceptance and being welcomed by others. *Global evaluations of self* included descriptions of the self as friendly/ likeable, optimistic, funny/witty, calm/easy going, a good listener, interesting/intellectual, kind/car- ing, and helpful. Table 1 shows the number of citations for each category. The coding manual used in the qualitative analysis is available from the authors.

Perspective

Table 2 shows the number of memories recalled from the different perspectives in each group. Memories classified as "neither" perspective were excluded from the analysis as the numbers were so small. Each memory was analysed using a separate chi-square. There were no group differences for

TABLE 1
Self-concept descriptions

Category	High socially anxious	Low socially anxious
Participation		
Active	14	19
Passive	9	11
"True self"		
Differences true self/ what others see	5	4
Acting contrary to feelings	4	0
Enjoyment of social situations	6	13
Confidence		
Confident	7	18
Not confident (shy)	13	7
Talkative/lively/outgoing	11	17
Stability of self		
Stable	11	9
Unstable	19	21
Factors affecting descriptions of self		
Type of situation	24	25
Others in the situation	7	3
Interpersonal variables	5	6
Importance of others' opinions		
Evaluation (negative/positive)	11	10
Acceptance	3	3
Global evaluations of self		
friendly/likeable	18	15
optimistic	1	2
funny/witty	6	6
calm/easy going	0	1
good listener	2	1
interesting/intellectual	1	1
kind/caring/helpful	2	2

The numbers of citations per category for high and low socially anxious groups.

congruent memories, time 1: $\chi^2(1, N = 59) = 0.82$, $p = .37$; time 2: $\chi^2(1, N = 56) = 0.23$, $p = .63$, or for the first incongruent memory, $\chi^2(1, N = 58) = 1.04$, $p = .31$. However, there was a significant difference for the second incongruent memory, $\chi^2(1, N = 58) = 8.88$, $p < .005$, $\eta = .39$: high socially anxious participants recalled more memories from the observer perspective than from the field per- spective, whereas the low socially anxious group did the opposite.

Memory age and valence could both have affected perspective. Overall, memory age ranged from the last 6 months to 25 years (86% were between 1 and 4 years old). Age was log trans- formed due to skewness and analysed using a 2 (social anxiety) × 2 (congruence) × 2 (order of recall) analysis of variance. There was a significant main effect of congruence, $F(1, 52) = 6.94$, $p < .01$, $\eta^2 = .13$, but no other main effects or interactions: largest $F(1, 52) = 2.25$, $p = .14$ for effect of time. For all participants, congruent memories were more recent than incongruent memories (con- gruent $M = 2.18$, $SD = 2.03$; incongruent $M = 3.02$, $SD = 2.98$). Memory valence was coded using a qualitative analysis (coding manual available from the authors). Low socially anxious participants recorded more negative incongruent memories overall (time 1: positive = 7, negative = 22; time 2; positive = 9, negative = 20) than high socially anxious participants (time 1: positive = 14, nega- tive = 14; time 2; positive = 12, negative = 14); $\chi^2(1, N = 112) = 5.05$, $p < .05$, $\eta = .21$. Separate analysis of valence in the two incongruent mem- ories showed a non-significant trend for the first memory, $\chi^2(1, N = 57) = 4.1$, $p = .057$, but no group difference for the second, $\chi^2(1, N = 55) = 1.33$, $p = .25$.

Memory vividness and the role of self-consciousness

Table 2 shows the mean vividness ratings for each memory. Vividness ratings were analysed using a 2 (social anxiety) × 2 (congruence) × 2 (order of recall) analysis of variance with public and private self-consciousness entered separately as covari- ates. There was a main effect of public self-con- sciousness, $F(1, 55) = 4.53$, $p < .05$, $\eta^2 = .08$, but no other main effects and no interactions: largest $F(1, 55) = 2.77$, $p = .1$ for the interaction between time and public self-consciousness. Overall, memory vividness was moderately correlated with public self-consciousness ($r = .31$, $p < .05$).

TABLE 2
Number of memories recalled in each perspective and vividness ratings

		Perspective			Vividness	
		Field	Observer	Neither	M	(SD)
Congruent						
Time 1	High	16	13	1	3.75	(0.79)
	Low	20	10	0	3.65	(1.27)
Time 2	High	19	10	0	3.55	(0.79)
	Low	16	11	3	3.65	(1.17)
Incongruent						
Time 1	High	16	12	0	3.70	(1.26)
	Low	21	9	0	3.65	(1.17)
Time 2	High	12	18	0	3.65	(1.14)
	Low	22	6	2	2.82	(1.29)

DISCUSSION

The main aim of this exploratory study was to investigate whether congruence with self-concept influenced perspective taking in memories of social events. In both congruent memories and in the first incongruent memory, the two groups recalled more field perspective memories. However, there was a clear group difference for the second incongruent memory, where high socially anxious participants remembered more observer perspective memories, whereas their low socially anxious counterparts did the opposite.

The results of this study are surprising and require further exploration. First, high socially anxious participants did not use the observer perspective more overall. Current evidence suggests that they are most likely to use the observer perspective in high anxious social situations (Coles et al., 2001) and participants here remembered a range of events that varied in both valence and mood, which may explain the absence of a general effect. We did not rate anxiety specifically and this would be important for future studies. However, the results do raise a question for current cognitive models of social phobia. Second, unlike Libby and Eibach (2002), we did not find a general effect of incongruence; instead we found a discrepancy between the results of the first and second incongruent memories, where high, but not low, socially anxious participants recalled more memories from the observer perspective in the second memory.

The discrepancy between the two incongruent memories is puzzling. Differences in memory age cannot account for it. Differences in valence may have contributed, but would be more convincing if

the group difference had occurred in the second rather than the first memory. Of course, the absence of an effect in the first memory may be due to a Type II error, or the result of participants failing to recall genuinely incongruent memories. However, if the results are not attributable to error, then we need to consider other possibilities. For example, the first incongruent memory may have primed the second, producing increased awareness of discrepancies between self-concept and the recalled event. Individuals with unstable self-concepts may be more vulnerable to priming effects than individuals with stable self-concepts. However, there is no direct evidence for this suggestion and it requires empirical testing.

It was also interesting that high socially anxious participants recalled both positive and negative memories in the incongruent condition. Further exploration of how memory valence affects perspective, and relates to different aspects of self-concept is needed. The results suggest that both positive and negative memories may trigger the "not me" phenomenon. Libby and Eibach (2002) argue that "not me" experiences occur when individuals remember behaviour(s) that no longer fit with their current self-view. This study indicates that "not me" experiences are not limited to past selves, but may occur in response to different aspects of current self-concept.

A subsidiary aim was to look at the concepts that high and low socially anxious participants use to describe their social selves. With the exception of references to the true self, participants did not differ in the range of concepts that they used, although the qualitative analysis of citations suggested that high socially anxious participants described themselves as less confident and more shy, as participating less, and enjoying social events less than their low socially anxious counterparts. The concept of a "true self" is interesting and further work, using both qualitative and quantitative approaches, is needed to explore how self-representations are made, stored, and changed. For example, do socially phobic individuals experience different kinds of self-defining memories from less anxious individuals? (See Conway & Pleydell-Pearce, 2000, for a discussion of how self-defining memories influence development of self-concept.)

We were also interested in differences in imagery vividness but found that congruence did not influence vividness, whereas public self-consciousness did to a limited extent. Public self-consciousness refers to awareness of observable aspects of self and to the impression that one makes on other people. This requires an ability to construct an inner representation of how one is coming across to others, and increased vividness may add to the perceived veracity of an image. This would be counterproductive if the image is a distorted, negative representation of self.

Individual differences in imagery vividness may explain the relatively modest correlation between public self-consciousness and vividness. Baddeley and Andrade (2000) argue that long-term memory influences imagery vividness by making sensory information stored in memory available, and by contributing to a meta-imagery judgement in which the individual decides whether the image could incorporate additional sensory information. Working memory also contributes by updating the image, thereby producing a sense of continuity, and by allowing the retrieved sensory information to be combined in novel ways. This model has important implications for social phobia. First, the sensory information derived from long-term memory may date back to specific aversive events (Hackmann et al., 2000), be distorted, and be attached to high levels of negative affect, for example, images associated with memories of being bullied. Second, combining information in novel ways allows the individual to construct a negative non-veridical image but, importantly for treatment, also allows the person to construct a new and more adaptive image. Precisely how these image formation processes interact with perspective is unknown and requires further investigation. Understanding these processes would greatly enrich current cognitive models of social anxiety.

The present study is a preliminary investigation and inevitably has a number of limitations. The median split used to form the groups may have produced less clear-cut results because scorers from the middle range were included in both groups. Replicating the experiment on participants selected for high and low social anxiety and on patients with social phobia would overcome this problem. The instructions used to elicit self-descriptions may have introduced a methodological confound by influencing the images that were subsequently retrieved. However, Libby and Eibach (2002) obtained clear effects for incongruent memories using a very similar methodology. The descriptions of self-concept were not controlled in any way, and although this allowed us to examine the themes that participants used to describe themselves, we could not draw any definite conclusions about differences between the groups. Future studies could combine a qualitative approach with more standardised personality measures or incorporate ratings of specific dimensions in order to increase comparability across participants. Finally, although we looked at the memories using a qualitative analysis, we did not do a manipulation check of congruence and future studies would be advised to include such a check.

The results of this study suggest a number of directions for future research. One critical question concerns how individuals construct a representation of self and what roles memory and perspective play in this process. Further work on imagery vividness is also important; for example, how does vividness affect the constructed impression? A more vivid image may demand more attentional resources, thus increasing self-focused attention and reducing attention to external feedback. Alternatively, if a distorted image is extremely vivid, this may increase the perceived veracity of the image. The role of memory and imagery in creating a distorted image of self is not limited to times when individuals participate in social interaction; memory and imagery also play a crucial role in anticipatory and post-event processing. Both of these processes are poorly understood and require further exploration. By answering these questions, we will be in a much better position to understand social phobia, and to help people to overcome it.

REFERENCES

Baddeley, A. D., & Andrade, J. (2000). Working memory and the vividness of imagery. *Journal of Experimental Psychology: General, 129*, 126–145.

Clark, D. M. (2001). A cognitive perspective on social phobia. In W. R. Crozier & L. E. Alden (Eds.), *International handbook of social anxiety: Concepts, research and interventions relating to the self and shyness* (pp. 405–430). Chichester, UK: John Wiley & Sons.

Clark, D. M., & Wells, A. (1995). A cognitive model of social phobia. In R. G. Heimberg, M. R. Liebowitz, D. A. Hope, & F. R. Schneier (Eds.), *Social phobia: Diagnosis, assessment and treatment* (pp. 69–93). New York: Guilford Press.

Coles, M. E., Turk, C. L., Heimberg, R. G., & Fresco, D. M. (2001). Effects of varying levels of anxiety within social situations: Relationship to memory perspective and attributions in social phobia. *Behaviour Research and Therapy, 39*, 651–665.

Conway, M. A., & Pleydell-Pearce, C. W. (2000). The construction of autobiographical memories in the self-memory system. *Psychological Review, 107*, 261–288.

Hackmann, A., Clark, D. M., & McManus, F. (2000). Recurrent images and early memories in social phobia. *Behavior Research and Therapy, 38*, 601–610.

Hackmann, A., Surawy, C., & Clark, D. M. (1998). Seeing yourself through others' eyes: A study of spontaneously occurring images in social phobia. *Behavioural and Cognitive Psychotherapy, 26*, 3–12.

Hirsch, C. R., Clark, D. M., Mathews, A., & Williams, R. (2003). Self-images play a causal role in social phobia. *Behavior Research and Therapy, 41*, 909–921.

Joffe, H., & Yardley, L. (2004) Content and thematic analysis. In D. F. Marks & L. Yardley (Eds.), *Research methods for clinical and health psychology* (pp. 56–69). London: Sage.

Libby, L. K., & Eibach, R. P. (2002). Looking back in time: Self-concept change affects visual perspective in autobiographical memory. *Journal of Personality and Social Psychology, 82*(2), 167–179.

Nigro, G., & Neisser, U. (1983). Point of view in personal memories. *Cognitive Psychology, 15*, 467–482.

Rapee, R. M., & Heimberg, R. G. (1997). A cognitive-behavioural model of anxiety in social phobia. *Behaviour Research and Therapy, 35*, 741–756.

Robinson, J. A., & Swanson, K. L. (1993). Field and observer modes of remembering. *Memory, 1*(3), 169–184.

Scheier, M.F., & Carver, C. S. (1985). The self-consciousness scale: A revised version for use with general populations. *Journal of Applied Social Psychology, 15*, 687–699.

Spurr, J., & Stopa, L. (2003). The observer perspective: Effects on social anxiety and performance. *Behaviour Research and Therapy, 41*, 1009–1028.

Stopa, L., & Clark, D. M. (2001). Social phobia: Comments on the viability and validity of an analogue research strategy and British norms for the Fear of Negative Evaluation Scale. *Behavioural and Cognitive Psychotherapy, 29*, 423–430.

Watson, D., & Friend, R. (1969). Measurement of social-evaluative anxiety. *Journal of Consulting and Clinical Psychology, 33*, 448–457.

Wells, A., Clark, D. M., & Ahmad, S. (1998). How do I look with my minds eye: Perspective taking in social phobic imagery. *Behavior Research and Therapy, 36*, 631–634.

Wells, A., & Papageorgiou, C. (1998). Social phobia: Effects of external attention on anxiety, negative beliefs, and perspective taking. *Behaviour Therapy, 29*, 357–370.

Wells, A., & Papageorgiou, C. (1999). The observer perspective: Biased imagery in social phobia, agoraphobia, and blood/injury phobia. *Behaviour Research and Therapy, 37*, 653–658.

Wells, A., & Papageorgiou, C. (2001). Social phobic interoception: Effects of bodily information on anxiety, beliefs and self-processing. *Behaviour Research and Therapy, 39*, 1–11.

MEMORY, 2004, 12 (4), 496–506

Negative self-imagery in social anxiety contaminates social interactions

Colette R. Hirsch, Tim Meynen, and David M. Clark

Institute of Psychiatry, London, UK

Patients with social phobia report experiencing negative images of themselves performing poorly when in feared social situations. The present study investigates whether such negative self-imagery (based on memory of past social situations) contaminates social interactions. High socially anxious volunteers participated in two conversations with another volunteer (conversational partner). During one conversation, the socially anxious volunteers held in mind a negative self-image, and during the other they held in mind a less negative (control) self-image. As predicted, when holding the negative image the socially anxious volunteers felt more anxious, reported using more safety behaviours, believed that they performed more poorly, and showed greater overestimation of how poorly they came across (relative to ratings by the conversational partner). Conversational partners rated the socially anxious volunteers' performance as poorer in the negative image condition. Furthermore, the conversation was contaminated since both groups of participants rated its quality as poorer in the negative image condition.

Individuals with high social anxiety fear that other people will evaluate them negatively. They think that this will occur as a consequence of them showing signs of anxiety, or behaving in manner that will embarrass or humiliate themselves in social situations such as public speaking, writing or eating in public, group situations, or talking to people they do not know. Social phobia is the third most prevalent psychiatric disorder, with estimated lifetime prevalence rates of between 7.3% and 13.3% (Kessler et al., 1994; Wittchen, Stein, & Kessler, 1999), with onset often in childhood or early teens (Schneier, Johnson, Hornig, Leibowitz, & Weissman, 1992). Individuals who experience high levels of anxiety in social situations often underperform at work and find it difficult to develop and maintain close relationships (Caspi, Edler, & Bem, 1988; Turner, Beidel, Dancu, & Keys, 1986). Social phobia can also lead to high levels of alcohol use, depression, and suicide (Schneier et al., 1992). Unlike some other anxiety disorders where the feared situations can often be avoided (e.g., fear of flying), people with high

social anxiety often have to enter anxiety-provoking social situations. Although clinical observation suggests that people with social phobia rarely receive explicit negative feedback from other people, left untreated, social anxiety tends to persist throughout adult life.

Clark and Wells (1995) proposed a model of social phobia which suggests a number of cognitive and behavioural mechanisms that might serve to maintain the disorder. A prominent aspect of this model concerns mental imagery. In particular, it is suggested that when in feared social situations, patients with social phobia experience excessively negative images of themselves and use these images to make erroneous inferences about how they appear to other people. Consistent with this suggestion, Hackmann, Surawy, and Clark (1998) found that patients with social phobia report experiencing negative images that involve seeing one's self as if from an external observer's perspective. The content of the images appears to be closely related to the person's feared outcomes (e.g., a bright red face with sweat pouring off their

Correspondence should be addressed to Colette Hirsch, Department of Psychology, PO Box 77, Institute of Psychiatry, De Crespigny Park, London SE5 8AF, UK. Email: c.hirsch@iop.kcl.ac.uk

The Wellcome Trust funded this research.

http://www.tandf.co.uk/journals/pp/09658211.html

DOI:10.1080/09658210444000106

forehead) rather than being an accurate portrayal of how they actually come across (Hackmann, Clark, & McManus, 2000; Hackmann et al., 1998). Hackmann et al. (2000) also reported that the image, which often comprises a number of modalities, is based on a memory of an earlier traumatic social experience (such as being bullied, humiliated, or ridiculed by others) and appears to represent the abstracted essence of how the patient perceives themselves in the memory. The memory was often of an event that occurred around the onset of the social phobia, but patients had often not made an explicit link between the event and the negative self-image. The image may be what Conway and Pleydell-Pearce (2000) refer to as "event specific knowledge" within the self-memory system, which, due to the threat nature of the traumatic memory, has been linked to information about themselves, but not its autobiographical knowledge base, thus explaining the lack of connection between the memory for the original event and the self-image. It seems that the memory of the aversive experience may be laid down in the form of an image of the social self and this is reactivated later in life when the person is socially anxious. This may be similar to traumatic memories experienced by people with post-traumatic stress disorder (Ehlers & Clark, 2000).

Although the studies by Hackmann et al. (1998, 2000) indicate that patients with social phobia experience images of the sort specified by Clark and Wells (1995), they do not show that these images play a causal role in social phobia. To do this, it is necessary to manipulate the images experimentally and show that the manipulation modulates features of the disorder. To date only one experimental study has investigated the role of imagery in the maintenance of social phobia. Hirsch, Clark, Mathews, and Williams (2003) asked patients with social phobia to have two conversations with a stranger, one while holding their usual negative self-image in mind and the other while holding a less negative (control) self-image in mind. Compared to the control condition, when participants held their usual negative image in mind they reported experiencing greater anxiety, rated their anxiety symptoms as being more visible, and rated their performance as poorer. An assessor, who did not know which image was being held, rated videotapes of the conversations. Patients underestimated their performance relative to the assessor. This suggests that patients based their judgements of how they appear on information that was not available to

other people, and this information may have included their self-image. In keeping with this, the patients' underestimation of their own performance was greater in the negative image as compared to the control condition; the negative image may have contained information that they were performing particularly poorly, thus potentially explaining the greater underestimation in this condition.

Clark and Wells (1995) also suggest that negative self-imagery increases anxiety and motivates the greater use of safety behaviours, which are attempts to prevent or minimise the feared catastrophes encapsulated within the image (Salkovskis, 1991). For example, if the self-image includes the person blushing, then they may cover their face with their hands in an attempt to hide the blush. Safety behaviours can be either behavioural manoeuvres (e.g., avoiding eye contact) or mental operations (e.g., mentally rehearsing sentence before speaking). Alden and Beiling (1998) found that when high socially anxious volunteers talked to someone they believed would make negative judgements about them, they reported spontaneously using more safety behaviours than people who believed that the other person's judgements of them would be more positive. Safety behaviours can often have the unintended consequence of making the person come across as distracted or preoccupied. Others may interpret this as a sign that the patient is not interested in them, or does not like them. In keeping with this, Alden and Wallace (1995) and Jones and Carpenter (1986) report that people with high social anxiety come across less well and are liked less when people first meet them, and that their friends find them less likeable, sympathetic, and easy to talk to. Hirsch et al. (2003) found that the assessor who rated videotape of the conversation observed more symptoms of anxiety and poorer performance when patients held negative images in mind, as compared to the control images, thus indicating that imagery can elicit changes in observable behaviours, rather than just being confined to introspective reports. It is plausible that the observable changes could be a consequence of more safety behaviours being used by patients when holding a negative image in mind; however their use of safety behaviours was not assessed.

The current study aimed to replicate and extend the findings of Hirsch et al. (2003), using a high socially anxious non-clinical population. Socially anxious volunteers participated in two conversations with another volunteer (conversational partner). During one conversation the socially anxious volunteer held a negative image in mind, whereas during the other they held a less negative control self-image in mind. The image was based on a memory of a social situation when they felt anxious (negative image) or relaxed (control image). In an extension to the previous study, a conversational partner, rather than an assessor viewing videotape, rated the socially anxious person's performance. If the conversational partner observes a detrimental impact of negative imagery on performance, part of the socially anxious person's feared outcome (negative judgements by others) may have occurred. In order to test Clark and Wells' (1995) prediction that negative imagery motivates the use of more safety behaviours, the study assessed whether socially anxious participants reported using more safety behaviours when they held a negative image in mind. Furthermore, the current study is the first to assess whether the social interaction itself is contaminated by negative imagery, for example by causing the conversation to flow less well or be less engaging. Clearly, if negative imagery does have a detrimental effect on either the other person's view of the socially anxious person, the social situation itself, or both, then this may influence the likelihood and nature of future interactions.

It was hypothesised that the negative image condition will be associated with higher levels of anxiety, greater use of safety behaviours, self-ratings of poorer performance, an overestimation of how poorly they performed (relative to the conversational partner), and the conversational partner observing poorer performance by the socially anxious volunteer, and that both the socially anxious person and their conversational partner would find the conversation was of poorer quality (e.g., flowed less well; was less engaging).

METHOD

Design

Volunteers with high social anxiety participated in two conversations with another volunteer who was not aware that the study related to social anxiety or imagery. During one conversation, the socially anxious volunteer held in mind their typical negative self-image, and during the other they held a non-negative control self-image, in balanced

order. After each conversation, both volunteers completed measures to assess the socially anxious person's performance and the quality of the conversation. The socially anxious volunteers also completed measures to assess their anxiety and use of safety behaviours during the conversation.

Participants

All participants were recruited through local universities and completed the Fear of Negative Evaluation scale (FNE: Watson & Friend, 1969), which distinguishes between people with high and low social anxiety. To ensure that participants in the social anxiety group had high social anxiety they were required to score 17 or above on the FNE at screening (a score shown to be associated with high socially anxiety, Stopa & Clark, 2001), but there was no restriction on the FNE score of participants who were allocated to be the conversational partner group. A total of 28 pairs of participants completed the study, but two of the socially anxious volunteers did not remember to keep the specified image in mind during the conversation and therefore their data were not analysed. Consequently, the social anxiety group comprised 26 (6 male) volunteers, and the mean score on the FNE on the day of testing was 23.12 (SD 4.51), with all continuing to score 17 or above. The conversational partner group comprised 26 other volunteers (14 male) and had a mean of 9.81 (SD 4.34) on the FNE on the day of testing. The conversational partners were told that the experiment related to conversations, but were not informed that the study related to social anxiety or imagery. The socially anxious participant and their conversational partner had never met prior to the first conversation.

All participants also completed the Social Phobia Scale (SPS) and the Social Interaction Anxiety Scale (SIAS; Mattick & Clarke, 1998) to assess social anxiety; the trait form of the State-Trait Anxiety Inventory (STAI: Spielberger, Gorsuch, Lushene, Vagg & Jacobs, 1983) and the Beck Anxiety Inventory (BAI: Beck, Epstein, Brown, & Steer, 1988) to assess general levels of anxiety; and the Beck Depression Inventory (BDI; Beck & Steer, 1987) to assess depression. As would be expected, the socially anxious group scored significantly higher on all measures of anxiety and they also had higher levels of depression, but did not differ from the conversational partner in age (see Table 1).

TABLE 1
Participant characteristics means (standard deviations in parentheses)

	Socially anxious volunteers		Conversational partner			
	M	(SD)	M	(SD)	t(50)	p <
FNE	23.12	(4.51)	9.81	(4.34)	10.85	.001
SPS	23.50	(13.78)	15.35	(10.58)	2.39	.05
SIAS	28.73	(10.93)	20.50	(10.34)	2.79	.01
Trait-STAI	50.50	(8.38)	40.19	(7.78)	4.60	.001
BAI	9.62	(5.63)	5.81	(4.68)	2.65	.05
BDI	10.92	(5.76)	6.31	(3.95)	3.37	.001
Age	21.92	(4.26)	22.50	(4.20)	0.49	ns.

FNE = Fear of Negative Evaluation questionnaire. SPS = Social Phobia Scale. SIAS = Social Interaction Anxiety Scale. Trait-STAI = Trait form or the State Trait Anxiety Inventory. BAI = Beck Anxiety Inventory; BDI = Beck Depression Inventory.

Materials

State anxiety. After each conversation, the socially anxious participants completed the state form of the State-Trait Anxiety Inventory (STAI: Spielberger et al., 1983).

Behaviour Questionnaire. This 14-item questionnaire assessed observable aspects of performance and anxiety, with high total scores indicating more visible signs of anxiety and poorer performance. All items were rated on a scale from 0 "not at all" to 8 "extremely". The Behaviour Questionnaire comprised 11 items which sampled three factors in Mansell and Clark's (1999) Behaviour Checklist: "positive behaviours" (e.g., "confident", "relaxed") plus the new items "friendly" and "listening"; "specific negative behaviours" (e.g., "sweating", "hands trembling") plus the new item "fidgeting"; and "global negative behaviours" (e.g., "uncomfortable", "awkward"). The internal consistency of the Behaviour Questionnaire is high (Cronbach's alpha = .93). The overall score was the sum of the items, with positive descriptors (e.g., positive behaviours) reverse scored, so that low scores indicated better performance. The socially anxious participant and the conversational partner completed the Behaviour Questionnaire in relation to the socially anxious participant's performance after each conversation.

Safety Behaviours Questionnaire. This 16-item questionnaire assessed the use of safety behaviours, with high scores indicating greater use of safety behaviours. It was adapted for this study from an unpublished Safety Behaviours Questionnaire developed by Clark and colleagues for use in treatment trials of social phobia. The internal consistency for the full Safety Behaviours Questionnaire is high (Cronbach's alpha = .80). Clark and Wells (1995) indicate that safety behaviours can be grouped into two sets. One set involves avoidance of engaging fully in the social situation (e.g., "avoided eye contact") and these may have a contamination effect on the social situation, since they may result in the person appearing uninterested or bored, thus giving an overall negative impression. Other safety behaviours are more concerned with impression management (e.g., "checked that you were coming across well") and may be less likely to have a negative effect on how the person comes across. In view of this distinction, the items on the Safety Behaviours Questionnaire were divided on an a priori basis into two sub-categories. The first sub-category, termed "avoidance", consisted of 10 safety behaviours that were attempts to reduce the person's involvement in the social interaction and had good internal consistency (Cronbach's alpha = .70). The other sub-category, termed "impression management", consisted of six safety behaviours that were attempts to convey a good impression to other people. This sub-category also had good internal consistency (Cronbach's alpha = .68). The socially anxious person completed the Safety Behaviours Questionnaire after each conversation by rating each safety behaviour in terms of the amount of time the behaviour was used during the conversation, using a scale that ranged from a scale of 0 "not at all" to 8 "all the time".

Conversation Questionnaire. This new 12-item scale assessed how the conversation flowed, how interesting it was, and the role the volunteers took in the conversation, for example, "there were uncomfortable pauses", "the conversation was odd", and "the conversation was interesting". The wording of half the items differed between the socially anxious version and the conversational partner versions of the questionnaire, to ensure that both volunteers rated the same aspect of the conversation. For example, in the social anxiety participants' version of the questionnaire the item was "the other person had to lead the conversation", while the corresponding item in the conversational partner version was "I had to lead the conversation". All the items rated the amount of time the statement applied to the conversation on a scale of 0 "not at all" to 8 "all the time". Positive ratings were reverse scored, and a total score was calculated, with higher scores representing a more critical appraisal of the conversation. The internal consistency of the Conversation Questionnaire is high (Cronbach's alpha = .83). The socially anxious volunteer and conversational partners completed the measure after each conversation.

Manipulation of self-imagery for socially anxious participants

Each socially anxious participant generated both a negative and a control self-image with order (negative first vs control first) counterbalanced randomly within the group. The negative image was the one that participants typically generated in anxiety-provoking social situations, whereas the control image was a less negative self-image. The image was elicited using a semi-structured interview used by Hirsch et al. (2003) and adapted from Hackmann et al. (2000). For the negative image condition participants recalled a social situation in which they had felt anxious, and for the control image condition they recalled a social situation in which they had felt relaxed. Once a memory was brought to mind, the participants closed their eyes and were asked a series of questions about how they looked and sounded, how they felt, and how they came across to other people. The image elicited on the basis of the memory of feeling relaxed was termed the "control image", while that based on the memory of feeling anxious was termed the "negative image".

Filler task for conversational partner

While the socially anxious volunteers had the semi-structured interviews to elicit a given image,

the conversational partner engaged in a filler task that was designed to limit their opportunity to anticipate the coming conversation or ruminate on the previous conversation. The task was completed in separate room from the image induction to ensure that they did not know an image was being elicited by the socially anxious volunteer. The task involved underlining all Ls, Ts, and 2s on sheets of paper with multiple letters and numbers printed on it. Concurrently, they listened to a taped story that included reference to a number of animals or characters and they listed each as it was mentioned in the story. The duration of the task depended on how long the socially anxious participant's image-eliciting procedure took. All conversational partners completed at least five pages of letter deletion and listed numerous animals and characters.

Procedure

Participants initially completed the FNE, STAI-T, SPS, SIAS, and BDI. The conversational partner completed the filler task (see previous section). The socially anxious volunteer was randomly allocated to hold either a negative or a control image during the first interaction. The procedure to elicit the first image was then administered (see earlier). They were then asked to keep this image in mind throughout the following conversation with the conversational partner whom they had not met before. The volunteers were instructed that they could discuss anything during the conversation, but they must not comment on the experiment. All participants complied with this request. Conversations lasted for 5 minutes. After the conversation, socially anxious participants completed the State version of the STAI (Spielberger et al., 1983) in relation to how they felt during the conversation. Both volunteers completed the Behaviour Questionnaire and Conversation Questionnaire, and the socially anxious volunteer also completed the Safety Behaviours Questionnaire and indicated whether or not they had been able to hold the image in mind during the conversation.[1] The second image was then elicited, followed by another conversation with

---

[1] As stated in the Participants section above, two socially anxious volunteers stated that they did not hold the image during the conversation and the data from these conversational pairs were not analysed. All other volunteers stated that they were able to hold the specified image in mind during the conversation.

the same conversational partner and completion of the measures, as above. All participants were paid for taking part in the study.

RESULTS

State anxiety

A mixed-model ANOVA was performed on the socially anxious group's State-STAI data, with Order (negative image conversation first vs second) as the between-pairs factor and Image Valence (negative vs control) as the within-pairs factor. The only significant finding was a main effect of Image Valence: holding a negative image elicited more anxiety than holding a control image, 54.96 (*SD* 8.84) versus 36.88 (*SD* 7.50), $F(1, 24) = 87.45$, $p < .001$.

Safety Behaviours Questionnaire

Socially anxious volunteers' Safety Behaviours Questionnaire data were analysed using a mixed model ANOVA, with a between-pair factor of Order (negative image first vs second) and a within-pair factor of Image Valence (control vs negative). The only significant finding was a main effect of Image Valence: higher mean scores in the negative than the control condition, 61.88 (*SD*

12.80) versus 44.04 (*SD* 16.01), $F(1, 24) = 19.14$, $p < .001$. Holding a negative image in mind was associated with greater reported use of safety behaviours.

Behaviour Questionnaire

Mean scores for the Behaviour Questionnaire are given in Table 2. The data were analysed with a mixed model ANOVA, with a between-pairs factor of Order (negative image first vs second) and two within-pair factors of Image Valence (control vs negative) and Rater (socially anxious vs conversational partner).

There was a significant main effect of Image Valence, $F(1, 24) = 79.26$, $p < .001$, indicating that the negative image was associated with poorer performance ratings, and a significant main effect of Rater, $F(1, 24) = 21.01$, $p < .001$, indicating that the socially anxious volunteers' ratings of their own performance was more negative than the ratings made by their conversational partners. There was no significant main effect of Order, $F < 1$. The only significant interaction was between Image Valence and Rater, $F(1, 24) = 15.58$, $p < .001$, which was investigated using post-hoc Bonferroni-corrected paired comparisons. Socially anxious volunteers' scores on the Behaviour Questionnaire were significantly higher in the negative than the control

TABLE 2
Behaviour and Conversation Questionnaires

		Image	
		Control	Negative
Variable	Rater	M (SD)	M (SD)
Behaviour Questionnaire			
	Socially anxious volunteer	29.65 (12.05)	59.62 (18.98)
	Conversational partner	23.04 (15.31)	35.65 (14.99)
Conversation Questionnaire			
	Socially anxious volunteer	32.81 (9.19)	48.12 (10.54)
	Conversational partner	24.62 (11.20)	35.58 (14.71)

Means and standard deviations of Behaviour Questionnaire (completed in relation to socially anxious volunteer) and Conversation Questionnaire scores for socially anxious volunteers and conversational partners.

image condition: 59.62 versus 29.65, $t(25) = 8.40$, $p < .001$. Thus, attempting to hold a negative image in mind led the anxious participants to believe that they appeared more anxious and performed less well. Similarly, there was a significant difference between imagery conditions for conversational partners' ratings, with the partner rating the socially anxious participant as appearing more anxious and performing less well in the negative image condition than in the control image condition: 35.65 versus 23.04, $t(25) = 4.16$, $p < .001$. The socially anxious volunteers had a more realistic assessment of their own performance and symptoms of anxiety when they are holding a control image in mind, since their Behaviour Questionnaire scores did not differ significantly from the conversational partner in the control condition: 29.65 vs 23.04, $t(25) = 1.74$, ns. In contrast, when the anxious volunteer held a negative image in mind, they rated themselves more critically than did the conversational partner: 59.62 vs 35.65, $t(25) = 5.66$, $p < .001$.

In summary, self-ratings and partner ratings were both worse when holding a negative image than when holding a control image in mind, indicating that there were observable effects of the type of imagery held on visible signs of anxiety and level of performance, as well as on self-perception. The socially anxious volunteers' underestimation of their performance and over-estimation of their observable symptoms of anxiety were greater in the negative image condition than the control condition, as indicated by significantly higher difference scores (socially anxious volunteer rating—conversational partner rating) in the negative image condition, as compared to the control condition, 23.96 vs 6.61, $t(25) = 3.79$, $p < .001$, consistent with the interaction of Image Valence by Rater reported earlier.

Additional exploratory analysis. Clark and Wells (1995) hypothesised that some of the deficits that other people observe in the behaviour of patients with social phobia may be a consequence of patients using safety behaviours. To assess this possibility, correlations were computed between the socially anxious volunteers' ratings of the extent to which they reported using various safety behaviours (Safety Behaviours Questionnaire) and the conversational partner's rating of the socially anxious volunteers' observable behaviour (Behaviour Questionnaire). As mentioned in the Method section, the Safety Behaviours Questionnaire was divided into two sub-scales, "avoid-

ance" and "impression management" on an a priori basis. The Behaviour Questionnaire consists of three factors ("positive", "global negative", and "specific negative"). As predicted, there was a significant correlation between the "avoidance" category of the socially anxious volunteers' Safety Behaviours Questionnaire and the "global negative" factor of the conversational partners' Behaviour Questionnaire, $r = .30$, $p < .05$, indicating that when the socially anxious person used more "avoidance" safety behaviours, the conversational partner observed globally poorer performance—however they did not observer fewer "positive" ($r = .17$, ns), or more "specific negative" ($r = -.029$, ns) behaviours. The "impression management" category did not correlate with any of the factors of the Behaviour Questionnaire ("global negative" $r = .07$, ns; "positive" $r = .17$, ns; "specific negative" $r = -.03$. ns), as predicted.

Conversation Questionnaire

Mean scores for the Conversation Questionnaire are also given in Table 2. The Conversation Questionnaire data were analysed using a mixed model ANOVA with a between-pairs factor of Order (negative first vs second) and within-pair factors of Image Valence (control vs negative) and Rater (socially anxious vs conversational partner). There was a significant three-way interaction between Image Valence, Rater, and Order $F(1, 24) = 4.83$, $p < .05$. Since there was an interaction between Image Valence, Rater, and Order, the Conversation Questionnaire data from the first conversation only were analysed with Image Valence as the between-pairs factor (control vs negative) and Rater as within-pair factor (socially anxious vs conversational partner). There was a significant main effect for Image Valence, $F(1, 24) = 16.88$, $p < .001$, due to higher ratings on Conversation Quality scores (indicating more critical evaluation of the conversation) when the socially anxious participant was holding a negative image, as compared to a control image (42.73 vs 29.38). There was a significant main effect for Rater, $F(1, 24) = 4.77$, $p < .05$, with the socially anxious volunteers being more critical than the conversational partners (39.35 vs 32.77). There was no significant interaction between Image Valence and Rater, $F < 1$. In summary, when the socially anxious volunteer held a negative image in mind it had a detrimental effect on the quality of the conversation for both the socially anxious participant and the conversational partner.

DISCUSSION

The results of the present study replicate and extend the findings of Hirsch et al. (in press). During separate conversations, socially anxious volunteers held a negative self-image or a control self-image in mind. When they held in mind the negative image, they reported feeling more anxious and believed that they came across less well (more signs of anxiety and poorer performance). Their impression that they performed more poorly was to some extent confirmed, since the person with whom they had a conversation observed objective changes in their behaviour and more symptoms of anxiety. Despite the observed detrimental impact on performance when holding a negative image in mind, the socially anxious participants overestimated (relative to their conversational partner) how poorly they came across and how evident their symptoms of anxiety were to a greater degree when holding the negative image in mind. Negative imagery was also associated with the socially anxious participant reporting more spontaneous use of safety behaviours, and both individuals found the conversation less interesting and thought that it flowed less well. The fact that the other person involved in the conversation observed this difference (or an assessor rating videotape, as in Hirsch et al., 2003) indicates that the feared outcome of negative evaluation by people with whom they are actually interacting may occur as a consequence of negative imagery.

Interestingly when the socially anxious person held a control image in mind, their own judgements of how they came across did not differ from the person with whom they were conversing, implying that under these conditions the socially anxious volunteer had a more realistic assessment of how they came across to others. This differs from Hirsch et al. (2003) who found that the assessor rated videotape of the patients with social phobia more favourably than the patient rated themselves, under both control and negative image conditions. It is possible that in its less severe form, socially anxious individuals do not underestimate performance across the board in the same way as people with the more severe form of anxiety, social phobia. Alternatively, the control image held by the socially anxious person in the current study may have been less negative and more realistic than those held by the patients reported in Hirsch et al. (2003), perhaps because, since they are less socially anxious, they could generate a more realistic non-negative image, thus enabling more realistic self-assessment in the current study.

It was only when a negative image was held in mind that the socially anxious volunteers' estimates of how anxious they looked and how they performed were significantly more critical than those of the conversational partner. The overestimation of poor performance relative to the conversational partner was over and above any objective changes observed by the conversational partner in the negative image condition. Given this, when holding a negative image in mind socially anxious people must be basing their judgements of how they come across on information that is not accessible to other people. As discussed in the introduction, Clark and Wells (1995) proposed that people with social anxiety might base their judgements of how they come across on the image itself, which contains negative social information (e.g., bright red face). Another source of internal information would be the anxiety they felt during the conversation. When the socially anxious participants held a negative image in mind they felt more anxious than in the control condition. Mansell and Clark (1999) have demonstrated that socially anxious people's judgements about how anxious they think they look are based in part on the anxiety they feel at the time. The increased anxiety reported in the current study may be a consequence of increased perception of social threat resulting from imagining the feared consequences of a social situation (i.e., looking anxious). Hence, the underestimation of performance when holding a negative image in mind may be due to the content of the image, the increased anxiety resulting from the image, or both.

Negative imagery also had a detrimental effect on the conversation itself, with more critical ratings of the conversation when the negative image was held in mind; both people involved in the conversation believed that it flowed less well and was less engaging when the socially anxious person held a negative image in mind. Although the conversational partner viewed it as less interesting and flowing more poorly in the negative image condition, the socially anxious person was consistently more critical of the conversations. This may be because they have higher standards for conversations in which they take part, in keeping with their high standard for their own social performance (Clark & Wells, 1995). A consequence of the social situation flowing less well may be that the person with whom the socially anxious person converses may not choose to seek the socially anxious person out for future social contact, thus providing negative social feedback.

As mentioned above, a further consequence of holding a negative self-image in mind was that the socially anxious participants spontaneously used more safety behaviours. As discussed in the introduction, when people feel socially threatened this motivates the use of cognitive and behavioural strategies that are adopted in that hope that they will prevent the feared catastrophe from occurring. The increased anxiety experienced as the result of holding the negative image in mind could have motivated the use of more safety behaviours. Data from Alden and Beiling (1998) indicate that increased anxiety is not a prerequisite for increased use of safety behaviours, since their volunteers spontaneously used more safety behaviours, despite not reporting increased anxiety. The content of the negative image may have provided the volunteer with information that they were performing poorly, and this may have motivated greater use of more safety behaviours to compensate. Hence, increased state anxiety associated with holding a negative image may have motivated greater use of safety behaviours, or the content of the negative image itself might have motivated the use of more safety behaviours in an attempt to prevent the imagined social disaster, or both.

The observed detrimental impact of negative imagery on the other person's assessment of how the socially anxious person comes across may have been the unintended consequences of greater use of avoidance-type safety behaviours by the socially anxious person. This is in keeping with Clark and Wells' (1995) prediction that one mechanism through which a negative impression may be given in social anxiety could be the unintended consequences of avoidance-type safety behaviours. The analysis conducted to investigate the relationship between the use of safety behaviours and the other person's impression of the socially anxious person provides some support for this idea. When the socially anxious person engaged more in safety behaviours that were attempts to reduce their involvement in the social situation, this was associated with the person with whom they were conversing generating a negative overall impression (e.g., more awkward) of the socially anxious person. There is an interesting paradox of the person with social anxiety engaging in safety behaviours that they believe will *reduce* the likelihood of their feared outcome occurring (i.e., other people forming a negative impression

of them), but these avoidance safety behaviours may actually *increase* the likelihood that their feared outcome will occur.

It is assumed that the effects reported in this paper are due to the person holding the negative image in mind rather than the control image. The control image was based on a situation where they felt relaxed socially. It could be argued that they may have generated an excessively positive image. This, however, seems unlikely given the close correspondence between self and conversational partner ratings of the socially anxious individual's performance in the control image condition.

The images elicited in this experiment were based on a memory of a time when the individual felt either anxious or relaxed in a social situation. The socially anxious participants were able to recall these situations, then focus on how they looked and sounded, any internal sensations they experienced, and how they felt emotionally at the time of the event. They then generated an image of themselves in the situation. The image often comprised different modalities (e.g., visual, auditory etc.) similar to spontaneously occurring images in patients with social phobia reported by Hackmann et al. (2000). It is noteworthy that people were able to generate an image on the basis of a memory and that this influenced their subsequent performance, behaviour, emotional reactions, and the flow of conversation. Furthermore, as discussed above, given the underestimation of performance in the negative image condition, the socially anxious participants appear to mistake the image for an accurate reflection of how they came across, as proposed by Clark and Wells (1995).

Research in clinical psychology often uses analogue populations, for example individuals with social anxiety, to investigate cognitive phenomena thought to play a role in maintain of clinical disorders such as social phobia (see Stopa & Clark, 2001, for discussion of this issue). Since the current study sought to investigate how social phobia's negative self-imagery impacts on social situations, it was appropriate to use a high socially anxious analogue population. However, it would be interesting to investigate whether requiring individuals without social anxiety to hold a negative image in mind during a social situation would have the same deleterious effects. Further research could be conducted to establish whether or not this is the case.

An issue that needs to be clarified is whether the extent to which the images were held in mind during the conversation differed between conditions. The current study assessed compliance with instructions to hold a specified image in mind during a conversation using a categorical variable ("Yes" the image was held, or "No" the image was not held in mind). This does not allow one to determine if the extent to which an image was held in mind differed between the negative and control conditions. Hirsch et al. (2003) used a dimensional approach to assess the extent to which the image was held in mind during the conversation, and found that patients reported that they were able to hold the negative and control images in mind to the same extent. Given this, it is possible that the negative and control images were held to the same extent in the current study, but further research will be needed to clarify whether or not this is the case for this high socially anxious population.

A clinical implication of the study is that social phobia may be alleviated by procedures that help patients not to generate negative self-images in social situations. In Clark and Wells' (1995) cognitive therapy programme, one of the main techniques for achieving this goal is video feedback, which can be remarkably effective at correcting distorted self-perceptions (see Harvey, Clark, Ehlers, & Rapee, 2000). Another technique for providing more accurate information about how one appears to others is to get patients to shift their attention externally and gather information about others' reactions to them. To enable patients to realise that even if they were to exhibit symptoms of anxiety evident in their self-image, people would not necessarily interpret this in the catastrophic manner they predict, surveys can be used where other people are asked questions about what they think of a person exhibiting a particular symptom of anxiety (e.g., blushing) and whether their opinion of the person would change. Another clinically useful technique involves the patient entering a social situation while exhibiting an exaggerated form of the feared symptom evident in the negative self-image (e.g., for a person who is bright red in the self-image, they would deliberately put blusher all over their face so that they look more red than is physically possible). The patient then monitors others' reactions to them very closely. This provides data showing that others do not react critically (if at all) to the symptom, and also enables them to realise that being in a social situation whilst exhibiting an extreme version of the symptom is tolerable. In keeping with the growing interest in restructuring early traumatic memories (Arntz & Weertman,

1999; Smucker, Dancu, Foa, & Niederee, 1995), the memory of the traumatic social situation, which may form the basis of the negative image, can be targeted therapeutically using imagery rescripting. Clinical observation suggests that this procedure can result in negative images no longer intruding spontaneously into consciousness. Finally, the procedure used in this study could help address negative self-images. Patients could be asked to recall social situations in which they felt relaxed and comfortable, and then elicit a non-negative self-image that they would hold in mind prior to and during subsequent social situations. The less negative image may be associated with lower anxiety, fewer safety behaviours, and better performance, which would be therapeutically helpful.

The current study experimentally manipulated socially anxious peoples' self-imagery and demonstrated that negative imagery contaminated the social situation in a variety of ways: negative imagery resulted in increased anxiety, poorer performance, greater underestimation of performance relative to other people, greater use of safety behaviours, and a less enjoyable conversation. People with social anxiety typically have spontaneously occurring negative self-imagery in social situations, this may serve to increase their anxiety, and result in a poorer impression being formed by other people and in the situation itself being less enjoyable for all concerned. This in turn could have the result that the person with whom they have interacted could be less motivated to interact with them in the future, thus providing a negative social experience, consequent on trying on ensure that a negative impression was not given.

REFERENCES

Alden, L. E., & Beiling, P. (1998). Interpersonal consequences of the pursuit of safety. *Behaviour Research & Therapy, 36*, 53–65.

Alden, L. E., & Wallace, S. T. (1995). Social phobia and social appraisal in successful and unsuccessful social interactions. *Behaviour Research & Therapy, 33*, 497–505.

Arntz, A., & Weertman, A. (1999). Treatment of childhood memories: Theory and practice. *Behaviour Research & Therapy, 37*, 715–740.

Beck, A. T., Epstein, N., Brown, G., & Steer, R. A. (1988). An inventory for measuring clinical anxiety: Psychometric properties. *Journal of Consulting and Clinical Psychology, 56*, 893–897.

Beck, A. T., & Steer, R. A. (1987). Internal consistencies of the original and revised Beck Depression Inventory. *Journal of Clinical Psychology*, *40*, 1365–1367.

Caspi, A., Elder, G. H. Jr., & Bem, D. J. (1988). Moving away from the world: Life-course patterns of shy children. *Developmental Psychology*, *24*, 824–831.

Clark, D. M., & Wells, A. (1995). A cognitive model of social phobia. In R. G. Heimberg, M. Liebowitz, D. Hope, & F. Schneier (Eds.), *Social phobia: Diagnosis, assessment, and treatment* (pp. 69–93). New York: Guilford Press.

Conway, M. A., & Pleydell-Pearce, C. W. (2000). The construction of autobiographical memories in the self-memory system. *Psychological Review*, *107*, 261–288.

Ehlers, A., & Clark, D. M. (2000). A cognitive model of posttraumatic stress disorder. *Behaviour Research & Therapy*, *38*, 319–345.

Hackmann, A., Clark, D. M., & McManus, F. (2000). Recurrent images and early memories in social phobia. *Behaviour Research and Therapy*, *38*, 601–610.

Hackmann, A., Surawy, C., & Clark, D. M. (1998). Seeing yourself through others' eyes: A study of spontaneously occurring images in social phobia. *Behavioural and Cognitive Psychotherapy*, *26*(1), 3–12.

Harvey, A. G., Clark, D. M., Ehlers, A., & Rapee, R. M. (2000). Social anxiety and self-impression: Cognitive preparation enhances the beneficial effects of video feedback following a stressful social task. *Behaviour Research and Therapy*, *38*, 1183–1192.

Hirsch, C. R., Clark, D. M., Mathews, A., & Williams, R. (2003). Self-images play a causal role in social phobia. *Behaviour Research and Therapy*, *41*, 909–921.

Jones, W. H., & Carpenter, B. N. (1986). Shyness, social behavior and relationships. In W. H. Jones, J. M. Cheek, & S. R. Briggs (Eds.), *Shyness: Perspectives on research and treatment*. New York: Plenum Press.

Kessler, R. C., McGonagle, K. A., Zhao, S., Nelson, C. B., Hughes, M., Eshleman, S. et al. (1994). Lifetime and 12-month prevalence of DSM-III-R psychiatric disorders in the United States: Results from the National Comorbidity Survey. *Archives of General Psychiatry*, *51*, 8–19.

Mansell, W., & Clark, D. M. (1999). How do I appear to others? Social anxiety and processing of the observable self. *Behaviour Research and Therapy*, *37*, 419–434.

Mattick, R. P., & Clarke, J. C. (1998). Development and validation of measures of social phobia scrutiny fear and social interaction anxiety. *Behaviour Research and Therapy*, *36*, 455–470.

Salkovskis, P. M. (1991). The importance of behaviour in the maintenance of anxiety and panic: A cognitive account. *Behavioural Psychotherapy*, *19*, 6–19.

Schneier, F. R., Johnson, J., Hornig, C. D., Liebowitz, M. R., & Weissman, M. M. (1992). Social phobia: Comorbidity and morbidity in a epidemiologic sample. *Archives of General Psychiatry*, *49*, 282–288.

Smucker, M. R., Dancu, C., Foa, E. B., & Niederee, J. L. (1995). Imagery rescripting: A new treatment for survivors of childhood sexual abuse suffering from posttraumatic stress. *Journal of Cognitive Psychotherapy*, *9*, 3–17.

Spielberger, C. D., Gorsuch, R. L., Lushene, R. E., Vagg, P. R., & Jacobs, G. A. (1983). *Manual for the State-Trait Anxiety Inventory*. Palo Alto, CA: Consulting Psychologists Press.

Stopa, L., & Clark, D. M. (2001). Social phobia: Comments on the viability and validity of an analogue research strategy and British norms for the fear of negative evaluation questionnaire. *Behavioural & Cognitive Psychotherapy*, *29*, 423–430.

Turner, S. M., Beidel, D. C., Dancu, C. V., & Keys, D. J. (1986). Psychopathology of social phobia and comparison to avoidant personality disorder. *Journal of Abnormal Psychology*, *95*, 389–394.

Wittchen, H-U., Stein, M. B., & Kessler, R. C. (1999). Social fears and social phobia in a community sample of adolescents and young adults: Prevalence, risk factors and co-morbidity. *Psychological Medicine*, *29*, 309–323.

Watson, D., & Friend, R. (1969). Measurement of social-evaluative anxiety. *Journal of Consulting and Clinical Psychology*, *33*, 448–457.

MEMORY, 2004, *12* (4), 507–516

A pilot exploration of the use of compassionate images in a group of self-critical people

Paul Gilbert and Chris Irons

Kingsway Hospital, Derby, UK

Self-criticism has long been associated with a variety of psychological problems and is often a key focus for intervention in psychotherapy. Recent work has suggested that self-critics have underelaborated and underdeveloped capacities for compassionate self-soothing and warmth. This pilot study developed a diary for monitoring self-attacking and self-soothing thoughts and images. It also explored the personal experiences of a group of volunteer self-critics from the local depression support group who were given training in self-soothing and self-compassion. Although using small numbers, this study suggests the potential value of developing more complex methodologies for studying the capacity for self-compassion, interventions to increase self-compassion (including imagery techniques), and their effects on mental health.

Self-criticism and shame have been proposed to play a key role in anger (Tangney & Dearing 2002), social anxiety (Cox, Rector, Bagby, Swinson, Levitt, & Joffe, 2000), mood disorder (Blatt & Zuroff, 1992; Gilbert & Miles, 2000; Gilbert, Clarke, Hempel, Miles, & Irons, 2004b), suicide (Blatt, 1995), alcoholism (Potter-Efron, 2002), post-traumatic stress disorder (Brewin, 2003), psychotic voice hearing (Gilbert et al., 2001), affect regulation and personality disorders (Linehan, 1993), and interpersonal difficulties (Zuroff, Moskowitz, & Cote 1999). Vulnerability to shame-based self-criticism is commonly rooted in *feeling memories* of the self being rejected, criticised, and shamed (Gilbert 1989, 1998, 2002; Kaufman, 1989; Tomkins, 1987), and/or abused (Andrews, 1998). Shame memories can be intrusive (Kaufman, 1989). Reynolds and Brewin (1999) found that depressed people often have intrusive memories of being shamed, rejected, and/or abused. Internalising these experiences can result in seeing and evaluating the self in the same

way others have; that is as flawed, inferior, rejectable, and globally self-condemning (Gilbert, 1998, 2002; Tangney & Dearing, 2002). Irons, Gilbert, Baldwin, Baccus, and Palmer (2004a) found a significant association between recall of parents as rejecting and low in warmth, and level of self-criticism in students.

When self-criticism emerges from a sense of a shamed self, people can feel beaten down and depressed by their own self-criticisms (Greenberg, Elliott, & Foerster, 1990). Indeed, intense self-criticism has been viewed as a form of internal harassment that is stressful and undermining of the self (Gilbert, 2004). Gilbert et al. (2001) explored self-critical thoughts in depressed people and malevolent voices in voice hearers, in regard to their "critical" qualities such as anger, intrusiveness, and the "felt power" of a criticism/attack. The study reported here expands on that methodology by piloting the use of a diary for self-critical people to monitor and report on the triggers and forms of their daily self-criticisms. A less

Correspondence should be sent to Professor Paul Gilbert FBPsS, Mental Health Research Unit, Kingsway Hospital, Derby DE22 3LZ, UK. Email p.gilbert@derby.ac.uk

We would like to acknowledge the enormous help of the Derby Depression Alliance Self-Help Group for their advice and participation in this study. We would also like to thank Rakhee Bhundia for her help with collating and analysing the diaries. This project was supported by NHS Executive funding.

DOI:10.1080/09658210444000115

explored aspect of shame-based self-condemning is the degree to which there is a relative *inability* to generate caring and self-soothing/reassuring, thoughts, feelings, and images (Gilbert, 2000a, 2000b). One source of self-soothing and self-reassuring is access to emotionally textured feeling memories of others who have been soothing and reassuring, e.g., loving attachment figures (Bowlby, 1969, 1973; Kohut, 1977). Mikulincer, Gillath, and Shaver (2002) found that threat can prime access to attachment inner working models and memories that are used for coping (for a review see Gillath, Shaver, & Mikulincer, in press). Irons et al. (2004) found that self-soothing and reassuring abilities in students were significantly associated with recall of parents as warm/affectionate and low on rejection.

A key problem for some self-critical people may be that they do not have access to feeling memories of being affectionately cared for (soothed), and their self-care abilities have been understimulated, underdeveloped, and underelaborated (Gilbert & Irons, in press). Some evidence for this was found in a study by Gilbert et al. (2004). They used an imagery task to explore how easy or difficult it was to imagine a self-critical/attacking part of the self, and a soothing, compassionate, and accepting part of the self. Those high in self-criticism found it relatively easy to imagine a self-critical part of self that was experienced as hostile, powerful, and controlling, while low self-critics found this imagery task more difficult. Self-critics found compassionate self-imagery more difficult, while low self-critics found this relatively easy to do. These data may indicate that self-critical people have more ready access to hostile self-to-self thoughts and feelings, and less automatic and easy access to self-soothing systems.

There is evidence that high self-critical depressed people may not improve as much as low self-critical depressed people in standard cognitive therapy (Rector, Bagby, Segal, Joffe, & Levitt, 2000). Helping people generate self-compassionate images and focus on feelings of warmth for the self may therefore be a useful therapeutic endeavour (Gilbert, 2000a; Gilbert & Irons, in press). Indeed, McKay and Fanning (1992) made self-compassion central to their cognitive behavioural approach for building self-esteem. Dialectic behaviour therapists also recommend developing compassion for the self (Linehan, 1993). Developing compassion for the self has a long tradition in Buddhist healing practice (Salzberg, 1995). Self-compassion differs from self-esteem in that it is focused on affects of warmth and sympathy directed at self (Gilbert & Irons, in press; Neff, 2003). In Buddhist practices, developing compassion for self and others can use highly structured images that are practised repeatedly (Dagsay Tulku Rinpoche, 2002; Ringu Tulku & Mullen, in press). The use of images to stimulate brain pathways for compassion may be powerful. For example, images have powerful emotional effects (Hackmann, 1998, in press) and are increasingly used in fMRI research to explore neurophysiological systems involved in certain kinds of memory, thoughts, and feelings (e.g., George, Ketter, Parekh, Horwitz, Hercovitch, & Post, 1995; Schwartz & Begley, 2002). To date, however, no study has explored how people might generate their own images of compassion to self, how they may try to imbue them with certain qualities (e.g., warmth and acceptance), and whether they find working this way helpful or difficult.

This pilot study did not aim to focus on the effects of giving intensive training in compassionate mind work, but to explore steps before that—to see how people experience their self-criticism on a day-to-day basis, to see what type of compassionate imagery they would be able to generate for themselves, and to explore whether they thought "practising self-compassion" could help counteract self-criticism. Clearly, one would have to think carefully about developing a psychological treatment that patients thought was inappropriate or unlikely to work.

There is increasing recognition that in investigating how patients may experience a disorder, processes associated with a disorder, or interventions, researchers should seek patient collaborative involvement in guiding and informing the research. Once patients understand what knowledge is sought they can offer insights from "the inside" (Goodare & Lockwood, 1999). Hence, given the nature of this research we recruited the help of a local self-help group for depression. The aims of this pilot study were:

1. To invite people attending a depression support group who have problems with self-criticism to take part in a collaborative research project investigating their inner self-critical and self-soothing processes.

2. To use a diary method to explore the triggers and forms (e.g., degree of intrusiveness and the power) of naturally occurring self-criticism, in this group of people.

3. To explore the ability to generate and use compassionate imagery, and obtain views of how helpful this may be for this group of people.

4. To explore the *types of images* generated and the experiences of working with compassionate imagery.

METHOD

Participants

A self-help depression group, with whom the authors have worked closely over a number of years, was advised of our study at one of their larger meetings. Those who regarded themselves as self-critical were invited to take part in this study exploring self-criticism and the use of compassionate imagery to help reduce it. Of the 18 people at that meeting, most expressed interest but 9 (2 men and 7 women) were able to take part and attend four $1\frac{1}{2}$ hour evening meetings. However, our data are based on eight participants due to incomplete data from one person.

All nine participants verbally reported that they had had at least one diagnosed depressive episode (diagnosed by a psychiatrist). All were currently on anti-depressants. All participants completed the Hospital Anxiety and Depression Scale (HADS; Zigmond & Snaith, 1983). The group mean for the depression subscale was 9.00 ($SD = 5.1$) and for the anxiety subscale was 11.83 ($SD = 3.6$). For the depression subscale, scores of < 8 indicate "non-cases", 8–11 doubtful/possible cases, and scores of 11 or above definite cases. One person scored 10, and four people scored 11 or greater.

All participants reported that they had had problems for longer than 10 years or "most of their lives". A number of participants had co-morbid difficulties such as social anxiety, agoraphobia, and obsessive-compulsive disorder. Our group was not pre-selected, other than that they attended a depression self-help group, they saw themselves as self-critical, and agreed to participate. Our focus was on self-criticism and imagery development rather than a specific disorder.

Self-attacking and self-reassuring diary measure

Diaries were constructed based on previous studies exploring hostile and compassionate self-imagery (Gilbert et al., 2004a, 2004b). They are available on request from the corresponding author.

We chose an *interval contingent* format for our diaries (Wheeler & Reis, 1991), which requires respondents to record their critical thinking over a set period of time. In this study, the set period was initially daily (for 2 weeks) and then weekly. Participants were asked to write down each day what situations or events triggered their self-critical thinking. Participants were also asked how these situations made them think about themselves, and how these thoughts made them feel. While Wheeler and Reis (1991) suggest that this method is open to retrospective bias, self-critical thoughts can often be variable in their frequency and duration, and can be difficult to measure using alternative diary methods. In the second section of the diary, participants were asked to give a quantitative rating of their critical thoughts and their ability to self-soothe in these situations, on a 1–10 interval scale. Ratings for self-criticism were given on: how often it occurred; how powerful, intrusive, long-lasting, distressing, and angry it was; and how difficult it was to distance from. This gave a possible range of 0–70. Ratings for self-soothing were given for how easy was it to: self-reassure, self-comfort, self-support, self-care, and self-soothe, giving a possible range of 0–50. As Ferguson (in press) points out, interval contingent diaries are useful when the subject being recorded is frequent, may not have a fixed start/end point, and may be continuous or sporadic.

Procedure

We arranged to meet with the participants for four evening sessions. During the first session, we outlined our interest in exploring with them the day-to-day nature of self-criticism, and how learning to be compassionate with the self, and focusing on compassionate imagery, might help to counteract self-criticism. The focus was to engage them as *joint partners* in this project. All participants agreed to the requirements in the spirit of a collaborative exercise, and signed consent forms that they were happy to take part. We agreed to have three consecutive weekly meetings, with a follow-up 4 weeks later. All participants were free to contact us if they had any distress associated with the procedure. None did, and in ongoing group discussion thought the process was useful.

Session 1: At our first meeting we discussed the nature of self-criticism. In open discussion, many participants thought that "a lot of this comes from childhood". Participants were asked to fill in various self-report questionnaires (not reported here) and to keep diaries of their self-critical thinking for the coming week. Instruction was given in how to use the diaries, with examples.

Session 2: Participants handed in their diaries and discussed how the previous week had gone. Following this, the first compassionate mind imagery exercises were conducted. This was introduced as part of training our minds to focus and attend to compassionate processes in the self (Gilbert & Irons, in press) in the following way:

> When we attack ourselves we stimulate certain pathways in our brain, but when we learn to be compassionate and supportive of our efforts we stimulate different pathways. Sometimes we are so well practised in stimulating inner attacks that our ability to stimulate inner support and warmth is rather underdeveloped. What we would like to do today is see if we can generate some compassionate images and ways of thinking that you can practise using over the next week and see how this may help you.

The group then discussed the nature of compassion, the value of compassion for the self, and key elements of compassion such as empathy, sympathy, warmth, and self-acceptance. The group had a discussion about whether developing these qualities for the self would be helpful, and the importance of training/practice in trying to generate these aspects for the self.

Following this, we engaged in imagery work. First, the group was taken through a short (3–4 minutes) relaxation process that focused on breathing and tension release. We then asked participants to imagine an inner place of safeness, which would allow them to do this work. They were then invited to "focus on an image of compassion that contains the attributes we discussed"; to "allow images to come to your mind that capture these qualities". Following this exercise, which lasted for about 10 minutes, the researchers asked each participant to share and discuss their images with the group. Participants were encouraged to practise their compassionate imagery as often as possible, and in particular to try to elicit it when they had self-critical thoughts. At the end of the session, participants were each given another diary to record their critical thoughts in the coming week.

Session 3: Participants handed in their diaries, and took possession of diaries that could be completed weekly rather than daily. As the next meeting was to be a month later, many felt it unreasonable to keep diaries each day for a month. We obtained feedback from participants on their experience of using compassionate mind techniques. We then took participants through the same process, again with the relaxation exercise followed by compassionate imagery practice, focusing on generating specific qualities of compassion.

Session 4: We met the group for the final time 6 weeks later. We had intended to meet earlier but holidays and other commitments prevented this. During this time participants were asked to keep weekly diaries of their self-critical thinking and abilities to be compassionate to themselves. Two participants were unable to come to the final session due to illness and child-care commitments. Again, we talked to participants about their experiences of using compassionate mind imagery, including specific aspects that they found helpful or difficult. A final form was given, asking participants five questions: What was the image that you have used over this research period? How did the image appear to you? What was the most difficult aspect? How much time were you able to practise? How helpful was it using the image? At the end of this session, participants were thanked for their time and help, and the researchers answered questions that were posed.

RESULTS

Triggers and forms of self-critical thoughts

Table 1 provides exploratory qualitative data based on the first three diary questions from Week 1 recordings. Two questions focused on types of thoughts and a third focused on what people felt as a result of what they thought.

Self-criticism was linked to a *multiple array* of activities and social interactions. In particular, many of the situations that activated critical thoughts were to do with relationships (including partner, family member, friends, and colleagues) and negative comparisons with others. Many self-critical thoughts were triggered by day-to-day occurrences, such as "housework", "visiting a friend", "given a gift from a client", "at the gym", "being awake at 3 am", and "having a headache". Also of interest is the wide range of critical thoughts and feelings reported about the self,

TABLE 1
Self-critical themes

Question 1: *What situations/events brought them about?*	Question 2: *What sort of things did you think/feel about yourself?*	Question 3: *How did your thoughts about yourself make you feel?*
Family	Inadequate	Inability to meet required standards
Visiting/socialising with friend	Incompetent	Unhappy
Given a gift	Angry	Anxious
Waking at 3am	Frustrated	Inferior
Having headache	Negative body images	Lonely
Relationships	Unattractive	Disliked
Work	Lack of control	Dejected
Housework	Irritated	Failure
Gym/body image	Lack of organisation	Hurting
		Weak

Examples of self-critical themes elicited from diaries over week 1 (pre compassionate mind training) "Looking back over today, please could you carefully think about any critical thoughts you may have had".

including anger, frustration, inferiority, and depression. Some people felt harassed by their self-criticism: "it was always there whatever I did". More comprehensive data for each participant are available from the authors.

Qualities of self-criticism

Alongside the qualitative diary information, we also asked participants to give quantitative ratings of their self-criticism (e.g., its power, intrusiveness, and hostility) and their ability and ease of self-soothing. Table 2 gives each participant's scores for baseline depression, self-criticism and self-soothing, and post compassionate mind training scores (after 1 week of practice) for self-criticism and self-soothing. We had hoped to obtain diary data from the fourth session to see how compassionate mind training had progressed over 6 weeks. Unfortunately, all participants had experienced problems in keeping diaries over this time (e.g., losing diaries, forgetting to fill them in) and so this set of data is unreliable. We would advise researchers to use shorter time periods or more frequent sampling points.

A paired t-test revealed the small reduction in scores for self-criticism was non-significant: mean score baseline = 42.35, (SD = 13.7) mean score post compassionate mind training = 37.46 (SD = 11.2); $t(7)$ = 1.32, p = .22. One patient who had been more self-critical in the week (participant 6) felt this was related to unforeseen life events.

Self-soothing

In regard to self-soothing/compassion, there was a significant increase in the ease of generating these images and soothing oneself in a self-critical

TABLE 2
Participant HADS depressions scores pre-training, and mean criticism and compassion scores pre and post compassionate mind (CM) training

Participant	HADS depression subscale score	Criticism pre CM training	Criticism post CM training	Compassion pre CM training	Compassion post CM training
1	5	46.57	22.85	19.25	30.87
2	0	38.18	39.53	24.33	32.50
3	16	56.50	58.25	5.00	12.25
4	13	64.50	46.77	7.00	20.32
5	11	44.86	39.50	12.71	18.84
6	10	22.43	28.73	29.14	29.00
7	12	34.88	32.68	20.00	20.00
8	7	30.91	31.40	7.17	6.40

situation: mean score baseline = 15.57 (SD = 9.0), mean score post compassionate mind training = 21.27 (SD = 9.2); t (7) = 2.94, p = .02.

Experiences of compassionate mind training

On the final meeting, we obtained data from six participants in response to questions regarding their thoughts and feelings about compassionate mind training. These are given in Table 3.

Participants' images varied greatly. Some individuals focused on personified images, whereas others did not. Most images were visual. Those who found compassionate imagery helpful described their images as having calming, soothing, and caring effects. Those who said they found it less helpful had found it difficult to bring an image to mind, hold it in imagination, and practise it. One participant found her "compassionate image" turning into the stomach of a well-rounded male who reminded her of her ex-husband, which made the experience unpleasant. Intrusive negative images, at times linked with memories, when one is trying to create a positive image can be distressing. In Buddhist meditation, should this happen the person is invited to let the image go and become gently mindful of the compassionate image again (Dagsay Tulku Rinpoche, 2002; Ringu Tulku & Mullen, in press). However, this lady felt that she needed to work through her anger towards her ex-husband.

We explored participants' images, focusing on different components of compassion. Sometimes an image would change with practice. Participants discussed how different blends of compassion components (e.g., warmth, acceptance) were more or less difficult. One participant said that he could imagine warmth, but not acceptance. This may have been related to unresolved hostility, and he seemed to hold a "Groucho Marx" belief that "I wouldn't want to be a member of a club that accepted me as a member". Some participants noted that it was difficult to hold a compassionate image, and that feelings of warmth or acceptance were often "only fleeting".

DISCUSSION

This pilot study explored the use of a diary to monitor typical elicitors of self-criticism and their qualities, such as their felt power, intrusiveness, and distressfulness, and builds on earlier work

(Gilbert et al., 2001). Participants felt their self-criticisms were automatic, powerful, intrusive, distressing, and difficult to distract from (Table 1). Participants felt able to keep the diaries, and found them revealing of just how much they did self-criticise. They suggested that diaries like this could be useful in helping people monitor their self-critical thoughts, although participants may not have been able to discriminate the various qualities of self-soothing and this requires further study.

A second key question concerned how easy or difficult it is for people to learn to generate and use compassionate feelings and images for the self. One participant found that her compassionate image changed into something unpleasant and she could not hold a "nice" image in mind. Another felt that images were difficult to generate or engage with. However, the other six participants felt they had benefited from their efforts, and two participants felt it had been a "great" help, although all thought they needed more help and support to practice, and more work as a group.

We found that there was a significant improvement in the reported ability to self-sooth. One cannot attribute this necessarily to the compassionate mind imagery work because participants also felt that working as a group and sharing their self-critical thoughts and efforts to be kinder to themselves had been helpful. Imagery work might be helpful in that it enables people to "carry their images" with them and use them outside a group setting. We would also suggest that therapists need to explore the functions of self-criticism and fear of giving up self-criticism (Gilbert & Irons, in press).

In Buddhist meditation, developing compassion for the self involves giving people specific images to focus on (Dagsay Tulku Rinpoche, 2002; Ringu Tulku & Mullen, in press). However, this pilot study was based on guided discovery and we were interested in how people generate their *own* images and work with them. Table 3 offers insights into the kinds of images created and how they were used. In discussion, some participants felt it might have been easier if they had been given specific images to focus on, while others thought they would prefer to work on their own images. For example, one person started with a religious image of a Buddha giving her compassion but could not make this "work" for her. She then generated her own image of a bush in bloom and found this very helpful. More research is needed in this area. We have no data on whether

TABLE 3
Full reported experiences of using compassionate imagery from the six participants at follow-up

Participant Number	Question 1: What was the image that you used over the research period?	Question 2: How did the image appear to you?	Question 3: What was the most difficult aspect?	Question 4: How much time were you able to practise?	Question 5: How helpful was it using the image?
1	Floating in warm sea Comforting sensation Sights and feelings	Visual Feelings Sound	Conjuring up image when needed	When needed	Recognising self-critical thoughts when they occur Diverting/stopping self-critical thoughts
2	White bush with comforting arms	Visual Sense of warmth	Concentration Stopping whirling thoughts	5 mins to all day	Focus on things and self not being bad Helps ease pain of being high/low Need to be alone to succeed
3	Rainbow Candles underneath instead of dark sky	Visual Nice feelings	Hard to get feelings Easier to get picture Used chanting to try and get image	Couple of times per week	Not yet achieved compassion with self, but may with more practice
4	Spiritual/Jesus Love/caring/ support In the air Sunset/stars/flowers/ mountains	All senses Visual Beauty of flowers, sky, sunsets waterfalls The love of friends Peace	Would find imagination impossible because it is unreality I would be living in an unreal world, unreal ideals Lying to myself, pretending – dangerous for me Enjoy daydreaming	Several times per day Whenever needed Situations where am giving myself put-downs, feel inadequate etc Pull up using compassionate mind – my spiritual friend – reality	Made aware how little I think about myself Changing thoughts round Would not have survived life without my Lord God
5	Sun Feeling of warmth	Visual Brightness Open space Warmth	Breaking lifetime's habit of feeling bad about self Lack of compassionate people around me Hard to conjure up image – felt remote and cold	Only occasionally	Relaxation aspect helped calm anxiety Aware of benefits of being compassionate but unable to do. Frustrated that unable to do it Hard to do with no support
6	Arm round my shoulders	Visual Sense/feeling of warmth	Image turned into stomach of well-rounded male. Brought back difficult memories of ex-husband	5–10 mins	Not at all All good destroyed by that (second) image

an image of "a person" with compassionate qualities would work better than these non-person images. On this more research is needed.

Some self-critical people may have few caring and soothing memories to call on (Gillath et al., in press; Mikulincer et al., 2002). Thus, the self-care and self-compassionate system may be underelaborated (Gilbert & Irons, in press). If people cannot utilise memories of caring others to be self-soothing, then an important research question is whether training people to generate self-soothing imagery is possible, can be helpful, and can be laid down as memories for subsequent recall. Lee (in press) has suggested that compassionate imagery can be directed to that of a "perfect nurturer" that has distinctive features including sensory ones. These features may aid the ease of accessibility from memory on subsequent occasions, in the context of self-criticism. Moreover, Lee has outlined how compassionate imagery can be helpful with people suffering from post-traumatic stress disorder, marked feelings of shame.

In regard to developing compassion for the self, participants agreed with one member who said, "this will take time as it is breaking the habits of a life time." A number of participants reflected that even as children they could not recall parents being particularly kind or compassionate to them, but more often cold or critical. Participants noted that "being kind" to themselves was not "something they were used to" and "at times it seemed strange" to them. However, all agreed that if they could develop compassion for themselves this would help them. Our research is clearly very preliminary given the small numbers, but suggests that some self-critical people can see the benefits of attempting to become more self-compassionate, can generate a range of varied images with different features, and find it a helpful process. Questions arise about personified and non-personified images, and distinctions between feelings of warmth, acceptance, and strength that are part of compassion but can also vary from person to person.

This study suffered from small numbers, and also the fact that participants did not keep their diaries adequately for the full 6 weeks. Nonetheless, as a pilot study it points to the value of diaries, especially for monitoring forms of self-criticism and self-soothing, the acceptability of this intervention for patients, and the indications that, with development, it may be a helpful intervention for some patients. Future research may focus on the following:

1. What are the most useful, distinctive features of compassionate imagery?

2. Exploring how developing and practising compassionate imagery may aid people who have few memories of others being compassionate towards them.

3. Exploring how development in the articulation and accessibility of compassionate images may reduce the influence of self-criticism and help alleviate various emotional difficulties associated with it.

4. Investigating how a compassionate image(s) may change with practice and the impact of such change on self-criticism and affect self-regulation;

5. How to build this process into an established psychotherapeutic approach, such as cognitive therapy.

REFERENCES

Andrews, B. (1998). Shame and childhood abuse. In P. Gilbert & B. Andrews (Eds.), *Shame: Interpersonal behavior, psychopathology and culture* (pp. 176–190). New York: Oxford University Press.

Blatt, S. J. (1995). The destructiveness of perfectionism: Implications for the treatment of depression. American Psychologist, 50, 1003–1120.

Blatt, S., & Zuroff, D. (1992). Interpersonal relatedness and self-definition. Two prototypes for depression. *Clinical Psychology Review, 12*, 527–562

Bowlby, J. (1969). *Attachment: Attachment and loss* (Vol. 1). London: Hogarth Press.

Bowlby, J. (1973). *Separation, anxiety and anger: Attachment and loss* (Vol. 2). London: Hogarth Press.

Brewin, C. R. (2003). *Post-traumatic stress disorder: Malady or myth?* New Haven, CT: Yale University Press

Cox, B. J., Rector, N. A., Bagby, R. M., Swinson, R. P., Levitt, A. J., & Joffe, R. T. (2000). Is self criticism unique for depression: A comparison with social phobia. *Journal of Affective Disorders, 57*, 223–228.

Dagsay Tulku Rinpoche (2002). *The practice of Tibetan meditation: Exercises visualizations and mantras for health and well-being.* Vermont: Inner Traditions International.

Ferguson, E. (in press). The use of diary methodologies in health and clinical psychology. In J. N. V. Miles & P. Gilbert (Eds.), *A handbook of research methods in clinical and health psychology*. Oxford: Oxford University Press.

George, M. S., Ketter, T. A., Parekh, P. I., Horwitz B., Hercovitch P., & Post R. M. (1995). Brain activity during transient sadness and happiness in healthy women. *American Journal of Psychiatry, 152*, 341–351.

Gilbert, P. (1989). *Human nature and suffering*. Hove, UK: Lawrence Erlbaum Associates Ltd.

Gilbert, P. (1998). What is shame? Some core issues and controversies. In P. Gilbert & B. Andrews (Eds.), *Shame: Interpersonal behavior, psychopathology and culture* (pp. 3–36). New York: Oxford University Press.

Gilbert, P. (2000a). Social mentalities: Internal 'social' conflicts and the role of inner warmth and compassion in cognitive therapy. In P. Gilbert & K. G. Bailey (Eds.), *Genes on the couch: Explorations in evolutionary psychotherapy* (pp. 118–150). Hove, UK: Psychology Press.

Gilbert, P. (2000b). *Overcoming depression*. New York: Oxford University Press.

Gilbert, P. (2002). Body shame: A biopsychosocial conceptualisation and overview, with treatment implications. In P. Gilbert & J. Miles (Eds.), *Body shame: Conceptualisation, research & treatment* (pp. 3–54). London: Brunner-Routledge.

Gilbert, P. (2004). Depression: A biopsychosocial, integrative and evolutionary approach. In M. Power (Ed.), *Mood disorders: A handbook of science & practice* (pp. 99–142). Chichester, UK: Wiley.

Gilbert, P., Baldwin, M., Irons, C., Baccus, J., & Clark, M. (2004a). *Evolution, relational schemas and the internalisation of hostile and reassuring selves: Their relation to depression*. Manuscript submitted for publication.

Gilbert, P., Birchwood, M., Gilbert, J., Trower, P., Hay, J., Murray, B. et al. (2001). An exploration of evolved mental mechanisms for dominant and subordinate behaviour in relation to auditory hallucinations in schizophrenia and critical thoughts in depression. *Psychological Medicine, 31*, 1117–1127.

Gilbert, P., Clarke, M., Hempel, S., Miles, J. N. V. & Irons, C. (2004b). Criticising and reassuring oneself: An exploration of forms, styles and reasons in female students. *British Journal of Clinical Psychology, 43*, 31–50.

Gilbert, P., & Irons, C. (in press). Compassionate mind training, for shame and self-attacking, using cognitive, behavioural, emotional and imagery interventions. In P. Gilbert (Ed.), *Compassion: Conceptualisations, research and use in psychotherapy*. London: Brunner-Routledge.

Gilbert, P., & Miles, J. N. V. (2000). Sensitivity to put down: Its relationship to perceptions of shame, social anxiety, depression, anger and self–other blame. *Personality and Individual Differences, 29*, 757–774.

Gillath, O., Shaver, P. R., & Shaver, P. R. (in press). An attachment-theoretical approach to compassion and altruism. In P. Gilbert (Ed.), *Compassion: Conceptualisations, research and use in psychotherapy*. London: Brunner-Routledge.

Goodare, H., & Lockwood, S. (1999). Involving patients in clinical research: Editorial. *British Medical Journal, 319*, 724–725.

Greenberg, L. S., Elliott, R. K., & Foerster, F. S (1990). Experiential processes in the psychotherapeutic treatment of depression. In C. D. McCann & N. S. Endler (Eds.), *Depression: New directions in theory, research and practice* (pp. 157–185). Toronto: Wall & Emerson Inc.

Hackmann, A. (1998). Working with images in clinical psychology. In A. Bellack & M. Hersen (Eds.), *Comprehensive clinical psychology* (pp. 301–317). London: Pergamon.

Hackmann, A. (in press). Compassionate imagery in the treatment of early memories in axis I anxiety disorders. In P. Gilbert (Ed.), *Compassion: Conceptualisations, research and use in psychotherapy*. London: Brunner-Routledge.

Irons, C., Gilbert, P., Baldwin, M., Baccus, J., & Palmer, M. (2004). *Parental recall, attachment relating and self-attacking/self-reassurance: Their relationship with depression*. Manuscript submitted for publication.

Kaufman, G. (1989). *The psychology of shame*. New York: Springer.

Kohut, H. (1977). *The restoration of the self*. New York: International Universities Press.

Lee, D. (in press). The perfect nurturer: A model to develop a compassionate mind within the context of cognitive therapy. In P. Gilbert (Ed.), *Compassion: Conceptualisations, research and use in psychotherapy*. London: Brunner-Routledge.

Linehan, M. (1993). *Cognitive behavioral treatment of borderline personality disorder*. New York: Guilford Press.

McKay, M., & Fanning, P. (1992). *Self-esteem: A proven program of cognitive techniques for assessing, improving, and maintaining your self-esteem. Second Edition*. Oakland, CA: New Harbinger Publishers.

Mikulincer, M., Gillath, O., & Shaver, P. R. (2002). Activation of the attachment system in adulthood: Threat-related primes increase the accessibility of mental representations of attachment figures. *Journal of Personality and Social Psychology, 83*, 881–895.

Neff, K. D. (2003). Self compassion: An alternative conceptualisation of a healthy attitude to oneself. *Self and Society, 2*, 85–102.

Potter-Efron, R. (2002). *Shame, guilt and alcoholism: Treatment issues in clinical practice*. New York: The Haworth Press.

Rector, N. A., Bagby, R. M., Segal, Z. V., Joffe, R. T., & Levitt, A. (2000). Self-criticism and dependency in depressed patients treated with cognitive therapy or pharmacotherapy. *Cognitive Therapy and Research, 24*, 571–584.

Reynolds, M., & Brewin, C. R. (1999). Intrusive memories in depression and posttraumatic stress disorder. *Behaviour Research and Therapy, 37*, 201–215.

Ringu Tilku & Mullen, K. (in press). The Buddhist use of compassionate imagery in Buddhist meditation. In P. Gilbert (Ed.), *Compassion: Conceptualisations, research and use in psychotherapy*. London: Brunner-Routledge.

Salzberg, S. (1995). *Loving-kindness: The revolutionary art of happiness*. Boston, MA: Shambhala.

Schwartz, J. M., & Begley, S. (2002). *The mind and the brain: Neuroplasticity and the power of mental force*. New York: Regan Books.

Tangney, J. P., & Dearing, R. L. (2002). *Shame and guilt*. New York: Guilford Press.

Tomkins, S. S. (1987). Shame. In D. L. Nathanson (Ed.), *The many faces of shame* (pp. 133–161). New York: Guilford Press.

Wheeler, L., & Reis, H. T. (1991). Self-recoding of everyday life events: Origins, types and uses. *Journal of Personality*, *59*, 339–354.

Zigmond, A. S., & Snaith, R. P. (1983). The Hospital Anxiety and Depression Scale. *Acta Psychiatrica Scandinavica*, *67*, 361–370.

Zuroff, D. C., Moskowitz, D. S., & Cote, S. (1999). Dependency, self-criticism, interpersonal behaviour and affect: Evolutionary perspectives. *British Journal of Clinical Psychology*, *38*, 231–250.

MEMORY, 2004, *12* (4), 517–524

The use of imagery in cognitive therapy for psychosis: A case example

Anthony P. Morrison

Bolton, Salford & Trafford Mental Health Partnership, and University of Manchester, UK

There has been a long tradition of studying imagery in relation to psychotic symptoms. Recent studies have suggested that imagery may be involved in the development and maintenance of psychotic symptoms (hallucinations and delusions in particular). Following a review of this literature, including work conducted by the author and colleagues, a case study is used to illustrate the clinical applications of this work. Working with images that were associated with persecutory delusions appeared to contribute to a reduction in distress, preoccupation, and conviction in relation to these beliefs, which were assessed using a standardised measure (PSYRATS). The implications for theory, practice, and future research are considered.

There has been a long history of interest in the relationships between imagery and psychosis (e.g., Cohen, 1938). Traditionally, this has examined the role of imagery in the development or causation of psychotic experiences, particularly hallucinations. However, recent advances in the field of anxiety disorders has led to the examination of mental images associated with the occurrence of psychotic experiences, and the role they may play in the maintenance of hallucinations and delusions and the associated distress. These relationships will be considered, and the clinical implications will be discussed and illustrated with a case example.

IMAGERY AND THE DEVELOPMENT OF PSYCHOSIS

Several early theories regarding the causes of hallucinations implicated imagery (e.g., Galton, 1883). Several more recent studies have found support for a link between the experience of hallucinations and increased vividness of mental imagery. For example, Mintz and Alpert (1972) found that patients experiencing hallucinations reported more vivid auditory imagery than a non-hallucinating control group. Another study found that for patients experiencing hallucinations (mostly in the auditory modality), the relative level of vividness of mental images was higher in the auditory modality in comparison with the visual modality (Boecker, Hijman, Kahn, & De Haan, 2000). Similarly, several studies have found a statistical association between self-reported vividness of imagery and predisposition to hallucinations in the general population (Aleman, Boecker, & de Haan, 1999; Morrison, Wells, & Nothard, 2002b). However, the findings in this area are equivocal, with several studies failing to find a relationship between imagery vividness and hallucinatory experiences (e.g., Aleman, Boecker, & de Haan, 2001), and Bentall (1990) concluded that the vividness of imagery hypothesis has insufficient empirical evidence.

There has been very little research conducted examining the relationship between vividness of imagery and delusional beliefs. However, Morrison et al. (2002b) reported a significant association between delusional ideation and vivid imagery in a non-patient sample.

Correspondence should be sent to Dr Tony Morrison, Department of Clinical Psychology, Prestwich Hospital, Bury New Road, Prestwich, Manchester M25 3BL, UK. Email: tony.morrison@psy.man.ac.uk

http://www.tandf.co.uk/journals/pp/09658211.html

DOI:10.1080/09658210444000142

IMAGERY AND THE MAINTENANCE OF PSYCHOSIS

In his cognitive theory of emotional disorders, Beck (1976) suggested that appraisals of events affect how people feel and, as such, can be responsible for psychological disorders. He explicitly suggested that these appraisals could be accessed through imagery. Several studies have demonstrated such images in patients with anxiety disorders (e.g., Beck, Laude, & Bohnert, 1974; Hackmann, Surawy, & Clark, 1998). Recent studies of imagery in people with social anxiety have also demonstrated that the spontaneous images associated with social anxiety are often associated with life events that occurred around the time of onset of the disorder (Hackmann, Clark, & McManus, 2000).

Recent cognitive conceptualisations of psychosis have also implicated appraisal as a central process (Morrison, 2001). On this basis, Morrison et al. (2002a) conducted a study examining imagery that occurred concurrently with the experience of psychotic phenomena (such as hallucinations and delusions) in 35 patients with a diagnosis of a schizophrenia spectrum disorder. It was found that approximately 75% of psychotic patients could identify images that occurred spontaneously in relation to their hallucinations and delusions (for example, having an image of the perceived source of a voice when hearing it, or having an image of being attacked when experiencing persecutory ideation). For those patients who were able to identify idiosyncratic images experienced in conjunction with their hallucinations and delusions, approximately 70% reported that their images were recurrent and that they were able to associate the image with a memory for a particular event in their past. The vast majority (approximately 95%) were able to identify specific emotions and beliefs that were associated with the images.

A variety of themes were apparent in the images reported by psychotic patients, including feared catastrophes associated with paranoia or persecutory ideas, memories of real traumatic life events, the perceived sources of voices or other psychotic experiences (such as passivity phenomena), and the content of the voices. These themes are illustrated with some examples from patients, which are shown in Table 1. Morrison et al. (2002a) also reported that some of the patients used their images as evidence to support their delusional beliefs or beliefs about their voices.

TRAUMA, PTSD, MEMORY, AND PSYCHOSIS

As noted above, imagery in psychosis is frequently related to traumatic memories. Post-traumatic stress disorder (PTSD) is a common reaction to traumatic life events, which involves symptoms such as intrusive or unwanted re-experiencing of the event, hyperarousal, avoidance, and emotional numbing (American Psychiatric Association, 1994). PTSD is extremely common in people with psychosis, both as a concurrent disorder (Mueser et al., 1998) and as a consequence of psychosis or psychiatric treatment (Frame & Morrison, 2001). Intrusive imagery of traumatic events is viewed as a defining symptom of PTSD (Brewin, 1998), and

TABLE 1
Themes of psychosis-related imagery

Theme	Examples from patients
Feared catastrophes associated with delusions	Being chopped up with axes Self being pushed into an oven Self being cut in two by man wielding large sword Being led away to prison by two large policemen
Memories of real traumatic life events	Self rocking in a psychiatric hospital Being assaulted
Perceived source of psychotic experiences	Neighbours in bedroom talking about me Spirits of friends and relatives surrounding head Man with beard shouting Image of black sphere of energy close to head
Content of the voices	Sexually abusing young girls Picture of sharp instrument stabbing someone

it has been suggested that trauma memories are inadequately integrated with autobiographical memory in people with PTSD (Brewin, Dalgleish, & Joseph, 1996; Ehlers & Clark, 2000). In this context, it is interesting to note that autobiographical memory has been shown to be impaired in patients with a diagnosis of schizophrenia (Baddeley, Thornton, Chua, & McKenna, 1996), and similarities in form and content have been noted between psychotic experiences and the intrusive phenomena that characterise anxiety disorders (Morrison, Haddock, & Tarrier, 1995).

Several authors have suggested that there is a subtype of schizophrenia that is trauma-induced (Ellason & Ross, 1997; Kingdon & Turkington, 1999), and many of the images reported by Morrison et al. (2002a) would be consistent with this view. Recently, Morrison, Frame, and Larkin (2003) have suggested that dissociative processes and metacognitive beliefs may contribute to the development of psychosis in response to traumatic life events. They also suggest that traumatic life events may contribute to the development of psychotic experiences, which evolve as coping or survival strategies as a result of positive beliefs about unusual experiences (for example, becoming paranoid as a survival strategy for avoiding further physical or sexual abuse, or hearing comforting voices following a trauma). In addition, they suggest that the failure to identify intrusions as being related to previous trauma may be a factor in some people developing psychosis, which typically involves making external attributions for internal events (Bentall, 1990). Brewin et al.'s (1996) theory would suggest that this would be more likely to occur if the trauma is represented in situationally accessible memory (SAM). Therefore, traumatic events, PTSD and memory processes may also be implicated in the experiencing of imagery in people with psychosis.

CLINICAL IMPLICATIONS

If imagery is involved in the development or maintenance of psychotic experiences, then clearly therapists working with psychotic patients should incorporate questions about imagery in their assessments, and the information that is obtained should be incorporated in their case conceptualisations (a working heuristic that is collaboratively developed between patient and therapist to explain the processes that account for the development and maintenance of their difficulties, which is used to guide the choice of intervention strategies). If such images are linked to specific beliefs, then using methods such as the downward arrow, with questions such as "what does having the image mean to you?" or "if that image were true, what would be so bad about that?" may help to identify unhelpful beliefs about the self, world, and others. Similarly, if psychosis-related images are associated with memories of past events, questions such as "does the image remind you of anything?" or "have you ever had any experiences that make you feel the same way that the image does?" may be useful in identifying relevant early experiences or critical incidents that will assist the development of a longitudinal formulation.

It is also likely to be important to be able to reduce the frequency of distressing images or alter the content or meaning of such images. Effective modification of persistent images can require specific imagery-related interventions (Hackmann, 1997). These can include modifying the ending of an image, introducing humour to the image, or having an adult self establish control in the image, and such interventions can be useful for people with distressing psychotic experiences. If patients are using the images as evidence for their beliefs about psychotic experiences (for example, believing that a voice is omnipotent, powerful, and omniscient because they have a concurrent image of God or the Devil), then an exploration of their beliefs about imagery may be helpful.

Interpretations or appraisals of images can be important in the maintenance of the distress associated with them. Metacognitive beliefs about the meaning and significance of mental images can be associated with emotional consequences such as fear, hopelessness, and anger (Wells & Matthews, 1994). For example, some patients believe that having an image of something means it is real or may be likely to happen (similar to thought–action fusion). In such cases, a metacognitive analysis of the relationship between imagery and the real world can be beneficial. These beliefs can often be disconfirmed using behavioural experiments, in which the patient concentrates on positive images, such as winning the lottery or having their favourite football team win by 20 goals to nil, and observes the results. It is also likely that imagery-based strategies devised for working with patients with PTSD may be useful for people with psychosis, enabling re-interpretation of intrusive experiences as input from memory rather than a current and real threat (Ehlers & Clark, 2000).

A CASE EXAMPLE

The utility of working with images that are associated with symptoms of psychosis will be demonstrated using a case example. Joe, a 30-year-old male, was referred for cognitive therapy for his paranoid thoughts (his identity and some descriptive details have been changed in order to protect anonymity). He met DSM-IV (American Psychiatric Association, 1994) criteria for delusional disorder, and had a 3-year history of paranoid delusions and ideas of reference, which had caused significant impairment to occupational and social functioning.

Case history and conceptualisation

At initial assessment, Joe reported feeling paranoid about being followed and kept under surveillance by a group of people that he did not know. He believed that these people wished to cause him physical and/or mental harm for unknown reasons, but thought it possible that they were after him because they knew of his previous criminal activities. Other current difficulties included increasing alcohol use in order to cope with the paranoid thoughts, anger about the conspiracy, social anxiety, and difficulties in going out.

His life history involved growing up in a residential care setting, with very little contact with his parents, and in which he received physical punishments on a regular basis. He also had some experiences of being bullied. After leaving residential care, Joe moved around frequently, and had several brief prison sentences for relatively minor criminal offences. While in prison, Joe was seriously physically assaulted, which resulted in admission to hospital. As a result of his life experiences, it appeared that Joe had developed beliefs about himself as being a vulnerable and unworthy person, and viewed the world as an inhospitable and dangerous place and other people as being untrustworthy and exploitative. He had also developed procedural beliefs about the importance of staying vigilant for threat and being suspicious of others. He also believed, possibly accurately, that being paranoid had kept him alive in prison.

His beliefs about being harmed made him feel very anxious. He would avoid going out if possible, and when he had to go out he would adopt various safety behaviours (Salkovskis, 1991) in order to prevent himself from being attacked, such as walking different routes to and from the shops and avoiding eye contact with people. He was concerned that the people following him all used white transit vans, so he was highly vigilant for these. He frequently had vivid images of himself being thrown into the back of a van and being assaulted by a group of people with a variety of weapons.

The case conceptualisation, based on a recent cognitive model of psychosis (Morrison, 2001), was collaboratively developed and is illustrated in Figure 1. Such case conceptualisations are an integral component of cognitive therapy, providing a working hypothesis regarding the development and maintenance of a patient's difficulties. The purpose of such a diagrammatic representation is to summarise the important aspects of a person's life experience that have contributed to the development of beliefs that may be implicated in their ongoing interpretations of events (for example, developing beliefs about personal vulnerability and the dangerousness of others in response to childhood trauma may lead to paranoid interpretations of ambiguous events). Cognitive therapy assumes that these appraisals of events contribute to the experience of distress (e.g., "Those people want to harm me" would make someone feel scared or angry, dependent on their belief system), and that the responses adopted in relation to these may contribute to the maintenance of problematic experiences and appraisals (e.g., becoming increasingly vigilant for interpersonal threat will lead to the detection of more ambiguous events).

The case conceptualisation is fluid, rather than static, and is developed collaboratively with the patient, who provides the information, suggests relationships between the factors, and gives feedback after testing out the hypothesised relationships in homework tasks. It guides the selection of treatment strategies (e.g., modifying unhelpful responses or examining the evidence for particular interpretations) and assists in the prediction of therapeutic difficulties (e.g., difficulties in trusting the therapist).

Intervention and results

Sessions 1 and 2 were used to conduct assessment and generate a problem list and basic maintenance formulation. In addition to the cognitive-behavioural assessment that elicited the information

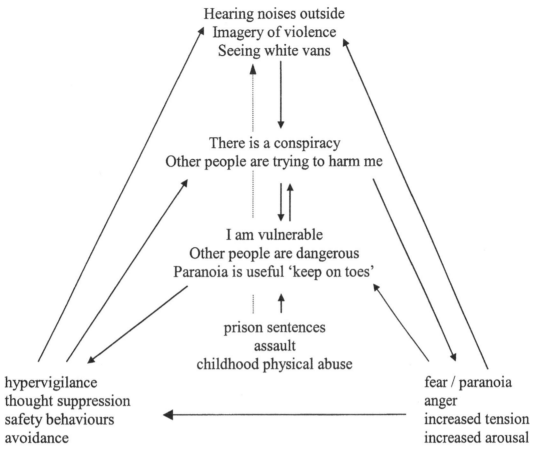

Figure 1. Case conceptualisation for Joe.

outlined above, Joe's paranoid beliefs were rated using the delusions subscale of the Psychotic Symptoms Rating Scales (PSYRATS: Haddock, McCarron, Tarrier, & Faragher, 1999), which is a six-item interview measure that assesses amount of preoccupation, duration of preoccupation, conviction, amount of distress, severity of distress, and impairment. Each item is rated between 0 and 4. The weekly results for the key dimensions of amount of preoccupation (how often the beliefs were experienced, ranging from no delusional beliefs to continuous or almost continuous pre-occupation), conviction (how much the ideas were believed to be true, ranging from 0% to 100%), and severity of distress (ranging from not at all to severe) are shown in Figure 2.

Sessions 3–6 involved primarily verbal reat-tribution methods such as examining the evidence for and against Joe's paranoid thoughts, con-sidering alternative explanations for incidents that he believed were part of the conspiracy (such as a white van being parked outside his house), and examining the advantages and disadvantages of

paranoia. As can be seen in Figure 2, his delu-sional beliefs reduced initially during this period, but then returned. Attempts were made to utilise behavioural experiments to test out his paranoid thoughts (such as going out without using his safety behaviours), but this was too threatening for him to consider.

In sessions 7 and 8, a collaborative analysis of his images about being attacked was con-ducted. The images were always the same, and involved being bundled into the back of a tran-sit van and then repeatedly being attacked with different weapons. These images were similar to an event that he had witnessed on televi-sion, but also caused the same feelings as he had experienced when he had been assaulted in prison, and to some extent resembled the assault in prison. Making this connection appeared to explain some of Joe's distress (to him), and his perception of control over the experience increased as a result. He decided to experiment with three different strategies for removing the power of the image: treating the

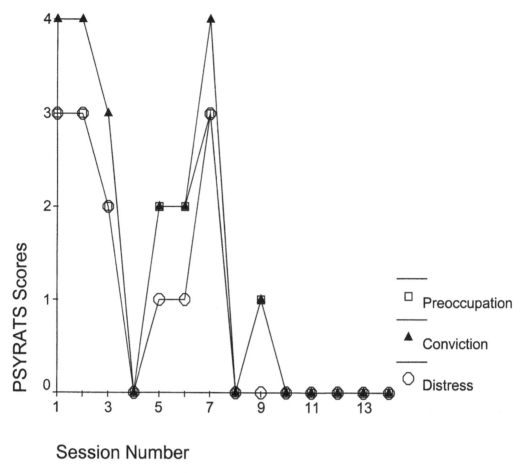

Figure 2. PSYRATS ratings.

image as a video (so he was able to fast forward, rewind, freeze frame, and eject it, and interrupt it with commercial breaks); introducing a rescuer to the image (his friends would turn up and chase away the attackers); and introducing humour to the image by incorporating his favourite cartoon character. He tried each of these in the session, and found a combination of the "video" method and humour (an interruption from an amusing advert) to be most successful in reducing his distress and increasing his belief that the image was only an image. This allowed him to feel sufficiently in control of the images to participate in behavioural experiments to evaluate whether or not he would be attacked if he went out. He also developed an alternative, safe image of being at home in front of his fireplace, in his favourite armchair, which he could utilise in order to reduce his belief in his thoughts and demonstrate that he could control the imagery, when

he was outside. These imagery-based techniques were practised as homework tasks and were used to facilitate subsequent behavioural experiments. The average ratings of distress, conviction, and vividness from the week in which he practised the use of safe imagery were as follows: belief in "I will be attacked" was 80% when experiencing paranoid images, and 0% when experiencing safe images; distress was rated as 62% and 25% respectively; and vividness was rated as 80% and 100% respectively. Figure 2 demonstrates that the focus on imagery coincided with a significant reduction in delusional distress, conviction and preoccupation, and that these reductions were maintained. The remaining sessions involved consolidation of the gains made in relation to paranoia, some work on social anxiety and self-esteem, and relapse prevention plans. These sessions also included a focus on occupational functioning.

DISCUSSION

It is evident that there has been a long history of interest in imagery and its relationship to psychosis. Whilst most of this interest has focused on the role of imagery in the development of psychosis, recent studies have examined the possible role of imagery in the maintenance of psychotic experiences and the associated distress. The application of imagery-based treatment strategies, and the use of imagery to inform case conceptualisations, has proved useful in the treatment of many non-psychotic disorders (Hackmann, 1997). Since most people with psychosis appear to experience recurrent images in relation to their psychotic symptoms, it is likely that the use of imagery-based strategies will also be helpful in the treatment of psychosis. In the case example presented, a lasting reduction in several dimensions of delusional beliefs appeared to be attributable, at least in part, to the use of imagery-based interventions. It is interesting to note that the images the patient experienced were similar to those experienced by patients with post-traumatic stress disorder. They caused similar emotions to his memories of a real assault in the past, but had been elaborated so that they were no longer identical to what actually occurred. As noted earlier, Morrison et al. (2003) have suggested that the failure to identify intrusions, such as vivid images, as being related to previous trauma may be a factor in why some people appear to develop psychosis, rather than PTSD, in response to traumatic life events. It is possible that such a weakened connection could be the result of a predominant SAM (Brewin et al., 1996). Making sense of the imagery in a way that incorporated life experiences appeared to be a useful strategy in this case, and could be conceptualised as changing from a SAM to a verbally accessible memory (VAM).

Clearly, this study only involved a single case, and further treatment research is required before a definitive conclusion can be reached; however, the single case design has been extensively utilised in clinical research. Future research should ensure a longer baseline period, and a more controlled application of verbal, imaginal, and behavioural intervention strategies would be desirable and should incorporate specific measures of dimensions of imagery. Additional research examining the relationship between imagery and the development of delusional beliefs, and the relationship between trauma, memory processes, and psychotic imagery is also indicated.

REFERENCES

Aleman, A., Boecker, K. B. E., & de Haan, E. H. F. (1999). Disposition towards hallucination and subjective versus objective vividness of imagery in normal subjects. *Personality and Individual Differences*, 27(4), 707–714.

Aleman, A., Boecker, K. B. E., & de Haan, E. H. F. (2001). Hallucinatory predisposition and vividness of auditory imagery: Self-report and behavioral indices. *Perceptual and Motor Skills*, 93(1), 268–274.

American Psychiatric Association (1994). *Diagnostic and statistical manual for mental disorders* (4th ed.). Washington DC: American Psychiatric Association.

Baddeley, A., Thornton, A., Chua, S. E., & McKenna, P. (1996). Schizophrenic delusions and the construction of autobiographical memory. In D. C. Rubin (Ed.), *Remembering our past: Studies in autobiographical memory* (pp. 384–428). New York: Cambridge University Press.

Beck, A. T. (1976). *Cognitive therapy and the emotional disorders*. New York: International Universities Press.

Beck, A. T., Laude, R., & Bohnert, M. (1974). Ideational components of anxiety neurosis. *Archives of General Psychiatry*, 31, 319–325.

Bentall, R. P. (1990). The illusion of reality: A review and integration of psychological research on hallucinations. *Psychological Bulletin*, 107, 82–95.

Boecker, K. B. E., Hijman, R., Kahn, R. S., & De Haan, E. H. F. (2000). Perception, mental imagery and reality discrimination in hallucinating and non-hallucinating schizophrenic patients. *British Journal of Clinical Psychology*, 39(4), 397–406.

Brewin, C. R. (1998). Intrusive autobiographical memories in depression and posttraumatic stress disorder. *Applied Cognitive Psychology*, 12, 359–370.

Brewin, C. R., Dalgleish, T., & Joseph, S. (1996). A dual representation theory of posttraumatic stress disorder. *Psychological Review*, 103, 670–686.

Cohen, L. H. (1938). Imagery and its relation to schizophrenic symptoms. *Journal of Mental Science*, 84, 284–346.

Ehlers, A., & Clark, D. M. (2000). A cognitive model of posttraumatic stress disorder. *Behaviour Research and Therapy*, 38(4), 319–345.

Ellason, J. W., & Ross, C. A. (1997). Childhood trauma and psychiatric symptoms. *Psychological Reports*, 80, 447–450.

Frame, L., & Morrison, A. P. (2001). Causes of posttraumatic stress disorder in psychotic patients. *Archives of General Psychiatry*, 58, 305–306.

Galton, F. (1883). *Inquiries into human faculty and its development*. London: Macmillan.

Hackmann, A. (1997). The transformation of meaning in cognitive therapy. In M. Power & C. R. Brewin (Eds.), *Transformation of meaning in psychological therapies*. Chichester, UK: Wiley.

Hackmann, A., Clark, D. M., & McManus, F. (2000). Recurrent images and early memories in social phobia. *Behaviour Research and Therapy*, *38*, 601–610.

Hackmann, A., Surawy, C., & Clark, D. M. (1998). Seeing yourself through others' eyes: A study of spontaneously occurring images in social phobia. *Behavioural and Cognitive Psychotherapy*, *26*, 3–12.

Haddock, G., McCarron, J., Tarrier, N., & Faragher, E. B. (1999). Scales to measure dimensions of hallucinations and delusions: The psychotic symptoms rating scales (PSYRATS). *Psychological Medicine*, *29*, 879–889.

Kingdon, D., & Turkington, D. (1999). Cognitive-behavioural therapy of schizophrenia. In T. Wykes, N. Tarrier, & S. W. Lewis (Eds.), *Outcome and innovation in the psychological treatment of schizophrenia*. London: Wiley.

Mintz, S., & Alpert, M. (1972). Imagery vividness, reality testing and schizophrenic hallucinations. *Journal of Abnormal and Social Psychology*, *19*, 310–316.

Morrison, A. P. (2001). The interpretation of intrusions in psychosis: An integrative cognitive approach to hallucinations and delusions. *Behavioural and Cognitive Psychotherapy*, *29*, 257–276.

Morrison, A. P., Beck, A. T., Glentworth, D., Dunn, H., Reid, G., Larkin, W. et al. (2002a). Imagery and psychotic symptoms: A preliminary investigation. *Behaviour Research and Therapy*, *40*, 1063–1072.

Morrison, A. P., Frame, L., & Larkin, W. (2003). Relationships between trauma and psychosis: A review and integration. *British Journal of Clinical Psychology*, *42*, 331–353.

Morrison, A. P., Haddock, G., & Tarrier, N. (1995). Intrusive thoughts and auditory hallucinations: A cognitive approach. *Behavioural and Cognitive Psychotherapy*, *23*, 265–280.

Morrison, A. P., Wells, A., & Nothard, S. (2002b). Cognitive and emotional factors as predictors of predisposition to hallucinations. *British Journal of Clinical Psychology*, *41*, 259–270.

Mueser, K. T., Goodman, L. B., Trumbetta, S. L., Rosenberg, S. D., Osher, F. C., Vidaver, R. et al. (1998). Trauma and posttraumatic stress disorder in severe mental illness. *Journal of Consulting and Clinical Psychology*, *66*, 493–499.

Salkovskis, P. M. (1991). The importance of behaviour in the maintenance of anxiety and panic: A cognitive account. *Behavioural Psychotherapy*, *19*, 6–19.

Wells, A., & Matthews, G. (1994). *Attention and emotion*. Hove, UK: Lawrence Erlbaum Associates Ltd.

MEMORY, 2004, *12* (4), 525–531

Images and goals

Martin A. Conway

University of Durham, UK

Kevin Meares and Sally Standart

Newcastle Cognitive and Behavioural Therapies Centre, UK

We propose that mental images are derived from goals. Goals are represented in a complex hierarchy and form a major part of the "working self". Images reflect the existence of specific goals and also act to maintain goals by facilitating the derivation of beliefs from the content of an image. Images in psychopathology may reflect the operation of dysfunctional goals: goals that are unconstrained and which increase discrepancy (experienced as anxiety) within the goal system. Another feature of the goal system is that it is conservative and avoids change. By this view some aspects of distortions in intrusive images of traumatic experiences might be viewed as a defence against goal change. Conversely generating new images might lead to the formation of new goals. These ideas are applied to the findings of the papers in this special issue of *Memory* and to several new case studies.

Conway and Pleydell-Pearce (2000) introduced a model of autobiographical memory that emphasised the role of the self and motivation in remembering. We believe that all human cognition is motivated but the goals that drive the system are processes that cannot be brought to consciousness. Instead the output of these processes in actions can be experienced and observed. Or mental representations can be derived from them, such as emotions, verbal statements, and mental images. In this article we argue that mental images have a special relation to goals. It is this relation that makes them so potent in maintaining dysfunctional states and also in doing quite the reverse—that is, in resolving such states. The papers collected in this special issue of *Memory* provide a unique source of fascinating studies that, at the very least, demonstrate the centrality of mental imagery in many different forms of psychopathology. Holmes and Hackmann have put together a fine special issue (for which we thank them), the aim of which is to stimulate thinking about the various roles of mental imagery in psychological disorders. It will undoubtedly achieve that aim and, as will be seen below, it certainly had that effect on us.

IMAGES AND GOALS

What is the function of mental imagery? Obviously mental imagery has several different functions. Here, however, we consider one central function, which is that mental imagery is a type of mental representation specialised for representing information about goals. It is a sort of "language" of goals. These might be goals relating to the future (e.g., social anxiety) or goals that influenced the past (e.g., PTSD). In either case when an image or set of images are in mind, important goal information becomes available and may influence current processing. For example, when a person who suffers from high levels of social anxiety brings to mind an image of a negative outcome in an interaction, then that image may itself increase anxiety and impair the current

Correspondence should be sent to Martin A. Conway, University of Durham, Department of Psychology, Science Laboratories, South Road, Durham DH1 3LE, UK. Email: M.A.Conway@durham.ac.uk

http://www.tandf.co.uk/journals/pp/09658211.html   DOI: 10.1080/09658210444000151

interaction (Day, Holmes, & Hackmann, 2004 this issue; Hirsch, Meynen, & Clark, 2004 this issue). A question that then arises is, why are goals mentally expressed and consciously experienced in images? In our view goals are *processes* (Conway, Singer, & Tagini, 2004) that cannot be directly or consciously accessed. Instead, representations can be derived from them and these might be in the form of images, emotions, or verbal statements. And, of course, they might be in the form of actions. Our suggestion is that images are highly associated with goals because they are close to actions. Indeed, they might in some instances and in some forms of pathology be mistaken for actions (Mansell & Lam, 2004 this issue; Morrison, 2004 this issue). Or they might have the same psychological status as actions (cf. Dadds, Bovbjerg, Redd, & Cutmore, 1997, and Dadds, Hawes, Schaefer, & Vaka, 2004 this issue) even though they are quite clearly not actions.

Consider, for example the following case of a person who watched the planes crashing into World Trade Center from a street close by. Two months later, very distressed, with an IES score of 36 (Horowitz, Wilner, & Alvarez, 1979; IES: Impact of Event Scale; a self-report scale commonly used clinically in the assessment of post-traumatic reactions. A score of 36 suggests a clinical level of impairment) he displayed marked avoidance and intrusive imagery:

> He had a powerful distorted image flashback in which he saw himself high above the ground observing the collision of plane and building. The scene is very peaceful and there is no noise. Whenever this, clearly false image, intruded into consciousness he felt intense, destabilising, guilt.

In therapy it was realised that this image meant marked avoidance of his emotional reaction, so in an early session he brought himself to ground in the image and remembered hearing the cries of the crowd standing around him and (finally) felt the anger and fear appropriate to witnessing the attack. Within a few sessions of working with this more realistic image his IES score was down to 10 and he formulated plans to return to New York to pay his respects to the victims.

Ehlers, Hackmann, and Michael (2004 this issue) provide many examples of the role of imagery in post-traumatic stress disorder and we will consider more of these and the "warning signal" hypothesis of Ehlers and colleagues further below. Here we might simply note that images in psychopathology often have the status of reality,

of actions, and this we suggest is because of their strong relationship to powerful personal goals. But note that dysfunctional goals, for instance avoidance of one's feelings, lead to dysfunctional images and this too is an issue we will return to below.

GOALS AND THE SELF MEMORY SYSTEM

Conway and Pleydell-Pearce (2000) proposed a mental structure they termed "the working self". A major component of the working self was a complex hierarchy of interlocked goals and sub-goals. This structure was considered to be permanently active with, at any given time, some subset more active than all other parts of the structure. The goal hierarchy of the working self modulates the generation of plans, actions sequences, and the encoding and retrieval of memories. Conway et al. (2004) extended the working self concept to include the "conceptual self", a set of beliefs, schemas, and models of the self derived from the goal structure and strongly associated with it. The working self and its knowledge base in long-term memory—autobiographical memory—together form the "Self Memory System" (SMS) and it is within this system that memories are generated and, we now suggest, images processed.

The relationship between imagery, especially visual imagery, and autobiographical memory is a powerful one. A diverse range of evidence (reviewed in Conway & Pleydell-Pearce, 2000) converges on the view that by far the majority of specific autobiographical memories are accompanied by visual imagery. Indeed, brain damage to areas known to support visual imagery can, as a secondary consequence, give rise to retrograde amnesia. This is because images associated with memories can no longer be consciously experienced.

One of the features to emerge most strikingly from several of the papers in this special issue of *Memory* is that images in several different forms of psychopathology derive directly from memories. Often these are memories of traumatic and negative experiences and also, of particular interest, patients are frequently unaware of the connection between their disturbing images and the memories from which they originate. May, Andrade, Panabokke, and Kavanagh (2004 this issue) provide strong evidence that imagery (visual and olfactory) is ubiquitous in the subjective experience of craving and desire. They also observed that imagery disrupts other cognitive processes. This is a property of specific autobiographical memories too (Conway & Pleydell-Pearce, 2000) which, when they come to mind, hijack cognition, turn attention inwards, and put the system into retrieval mode (Tulving, 1983). In the *elaborated intrusion* model of May et al., cravers create mental images of the desired state or object and this is pleasurable. In a similar way vivid images correlate with aversive behaviour (Dadds et al., 2004 this issue) and may even substitute for external stimuli in (aversive) learning sequences (Dadds et al., 1997).

Within the SMS model, images derived from experience or generated in other ways all correspond to goals. In particular they correspond to the ideal, standard, or referent in negative and positive feedback loops (Carver & Scheier, 1982, 1998, 1999). In a negative feedback loop the referent might represent a state of the world that is to be achieved or approximated to, and plans are generated that attempt to reduce the discrepancy between the standard and the perceived state of the world—in the SMS model goals and their sub-goals are conceived of as largely being a complex hierarchy of interlocking negative feedback loops that motivate cognition, emotion, and action. In this model images are representations of goal standards. Autobiographical knowledge and specific episodic memories (cf. Conway, 2001), are records of subsets of states of the working self goal system and so images deriving from specific memories are also of goal standards.

Thus the negative images that Hirsch et al. (2004 this issue) reported in patients with high social anxiety and those reported by Day et al. (2004 this issue) in agoraphobic patients were found to derive from memories of negative social experiences, e.g., being bullied, social humiliation, intimidation, etc. Similarly, the body dysmorphic patients of Osman, Cooper, Hackmann, and Veale (2004 this issue) had negative appearance-related images that were strongly related to memories of negative childhood experiences. And the self-critical patients studied by Gilbert and Irons (2004 this issue) had what they called "feeling memories" of experiences of rejection, shame, and abuse, from which derived severe internal self-criticisms. Presumably all these memories, and the images that come from them, represent states of the world that are to be avoided (Dadds et al., 2004 this issue) and may

then be derived from positive rather than negative feedback loops. Positive feedback loops (see Carver & Scheier, 1998, Chapter 2) have plans that aim to avoid a particular referent or state of the world, i.e., being bullied or intimidated. These discrepancy-enhancing goals are experienced by the individual as images and memories.

One interesting question here is why these images exert such a powerful effect on the individual. Why do they induce social anxiety? Why do they apparently maintain and intensify agoraphobia, body dysmorphic disorder, and self-criticisms? The SMS model with its emphasis on motivated cognition and the goal system of the working self suggests the following account. Memories of negative experiences form the referents of positive feedback loops in the working self goal-hierarchy. An important feature of positive feedback loops is that they are unstable in the sense that they have no boundary—the goal they represent is simply to avoid as far as possible the state of the world represented in their referent. In many systems positive feedback loops are bounded by negative feedback loops. For example as the distance increases from something that is to be avoided it eventually approximates to a value in a negative feedback loop. The discrepancy-reducing negative feedback loop might have as its referent an optimal distance from the to-be-avoided object or state. This might be experienced by the individual as a visual image of an actual state of the world, e.g., being at least two metres from a snake or spider. Images in social phobia, agoraphobia, body dysmorphia, and self-criticisms, might all then derive from referents in positive feedback systems that evolved out of early experiences, and which derive from memories of those experiences. The important point being that in psychopathology these discrepancy-enhancing systems are not bounded or constrained by discrepancy-reducing systems as they, perhaps, are in nonpathological cognition.

An important point to arise from this account of the goals of the working self system and their expression in images and memories is that if unbounded positive feedback systems can be constrained by negative feedback systems, then perhaps negative emotions and cognitions can be reduced. The promising treatment attempts described in these papers might be conceptualised as attempts to bound discrepancy-enhancing goals with discrepancy-reducing goals. It is especially interesting that this appears to be most effective if new images associated with positive affect, or positively toned memories, are formed and become linked in some way to the negative discrepancy-seeking cognitions. Repeatedly forming an image of the self may be a way of adopting new goals or of attaching to undesirable goal referents new desirable referents. An additional point here is that within the SMS model goal processing is considered to give rise to emotions (cf. Oatley, 1992). Emotions are ways in which the individual experiences progress in goal processing and they are also, like images, an impetus to action. Adopting new self-enhancing images, which become goal-referents, should then also act to increase positively toned feelings and the experiments by Hirsch and colleagues, and Gilbert and Irons, and the data from Day et al., all suggest that this may indeed turn out to be the case.

MEMORIES FOR TRAUMA AND THE PSYCHOLOGICAL DEFENCE AGAINST CHANGE

Ehlers et al. (2004 this issue) provide a particularly interesting set of case studies that illustrate various aspects of their theoretical conception of the nature and function of intrusive memories in post-traumatic stress disorder, PTSD (see Ehlers & Clark, 2000). Conway and Pleydell-Pearce (2000) provide a similar account, but from the perspective of the SMS model and with an emphasis on working self goal processing. In this section we extend our account to some new case studies of PTSD and attempt to link it to the Ehlers and Clark model and to the valuable case studies Ehlers et al. report in their paper. In agreement with Ehlers and colleagues we believe that trauma experiences often fall outside the range of the working self goal system. That is to say, that cannot be easily processed by the working self because they usually threaten the entire goal-system. Because of this the experience cannot be integrated with pre-existing autobiographical knowledge. But if this is the case, how then are such vivid and intrusive memories encoded?

Conway and Pleydell-Pearce (2000) argue that rather than being integrated with long-term autobiographical knowledge, PTSD memories are encoded in direct association with the working self goal structure and in particular with those parts of the system they most directly threaten. In the SMS model autobiographical memories are viewed as consisting of two types of knowledge: episodic memories and conceptual autobiographical

knowledge. Episodic memories contain sensory-perceptual knowledge that is experience-near and this is most frequently in the form of visual images (Conway, 2001). Autobiographical knowledge represents conceptual knowledge about one's life, e.g., about others, activities, locations, periods of extended activities, evaluations of lifetime periods, and knowledge derived from goals, etc. (Conway & Pleydell-Pearce, 2000; Conway et al., 2004). Autobiographical knowledge contextualises episodic memories and is always present when these memories are brought to mind. Indeed, episodic memories are usually accessed through conceptual autobiographical knowledge. There are, however, two exceptions to this. The first are very early childhood memories, which often seem to be fragmentary and have little in the way of a conceptual context, and the second are PTSD memories, which because they are unintegrated with autobiographical knowledge in long-term memory but are strongly associated to current goals remain highly accessible. It is, perhaps, not until the goal structure of the working self changes that these memories can become integrated with the knowledge base and so be rendered less intrusive.

Trauma memories are, however, destabilising because they provide information about experiences in which the goal system, or some significant part of it, was threatened. They are also highly accessible. According to the present account they will be activated and have the potential to enter consciousness each time the associated goals are activated, which probably occurs frequently. They are also highly accessible to cues encountered in the environment (Ehlers et al., 2004 this issue, provide many very clear examples) and this is because they are not embedded in autobiographical memory knowledge structures that would act to attenuate direct access to episodic memories by a cue. These highly accessible destabilising memories have to be defended against. We believe they have to be defended against because ultimately they require goal change, perhaps radical goal change. Conway et al. (2004) propose that goal change is particularly difficult to bring about, possibly because of the cognitive and emotional costs, and because changing one set of goals will have consequences for many other goals. Thus, at the heart of the goal system is a principle of conservatism that operates to avoid change.

According to Conway et al. (2004) the working self attempts to maintain the coherence of the self, and will bring about inhibition and distortion of episodic memories if these threaten stability. Ehlers et al. make the important observation that PTSD memories typically consist of several vivid details, of particular moments known as "hotspots" (Grey, Young, & Holmes, 2002; Holmes, Grey, & Young, in press) often surrounded by amnesic gaps, and these intrude into memory as "warning signals" related to moments of intense threat during the trauma. We would add to this that these image-based "warning signals" are also warning of the need for immanent and major change to the goal system if it is to survive the traumatic experience. Ehlers et al. (2004 this issue) also give several examples of memory distortions in PTSD. We suggest that the distortions in PTSD often (but not necessarily always) serve to protect the working self from the perception of the need for change. Consider the following case:

> A man who drove cars for a living was involved in a road traffic accident. He was a back seat passenger in a car when it was in a high speed collision with another vehicle; activation of the air bags in the front of the car produced a cloud of powder, which he thought at the time was smoke. At the time he could smell petrol and thought the car might ignite and remembers thinking "I will be burned alive." His wife was unconscious after the impact and he thought that she had died. He remembered thinking to himself "what am I going to do now?" as he thought about his future alone without his wife. He subsequently experienced intense guilt about this as it suggested to him that he was a selfish person. In addition, he was a very experienced driver and had anticipated the crash, but failed to cry out a warning. He felt that he could have averted the crash if he had done this. He experienced intrusive thoughts, such as "I should have shouted" (to warn the driver) and he relived the feeling of guilt he felt when he thought his wife had died, which he believed to be his fault because he did not shout out.

In this case the intense guilt and anxiety experienced when he recalled his failure to shout out was destabilising. So much so that daily activities were disrupted. During therapy—which included imaginal reliving of the trauma and a visit to the crash site—it became apparent that the way in which the accident occurred (the speed and orientation of the vehicles and their very rapid collision) meant that there could not possibly have been sufficient time to shout a warning. Once this *time expansion* distortion in the flashback was recognised, the intrusiveness and associated experience of guilt and anxiety diminished. The distortion then maintained the belief that he had in fact been in control and could have prevented the accident, when in reality this was not the case. What this patient had to accept was that despite his professionalism (a major part of his goal system) he was not always in control when driving.

The need to protect the self from change by distorting images in memories can also help maintain dysfunctional beliefs, such as "I was at fault", "I was the guilty one". A final case illustrates this quite strikingly.

> A 38-year-old man presented to the Borderline Disorder Therapy service with chronic self-hatred, a feeling of emptiness and impulsivity. For the previous 3 years, he had been unemployed and had done very little apart from hiding in his bed-sit and smoking large amounts of cannabis. He was referred for cognitive therapy following successful attendance at an educational group workshop on borderline personality disorder. Before this, he had led a chaotic life marked by impulsive relationships. In his early history, he described chronic sexual abuse from his grandfather, who had acted as his baby sitter as his parents worked very long hours as publicans. He remembers being abused from a very young age until the age of 12 when he was physically strong enough to retaliate. He never told his parents, as his grandfather threatened him that he would be taken away if he disclosed. He always felt different from other children as he was "soiled". As he got older, he would get sexually aroused when his grandfather was abusing him, which he took to mean he was at fault and an equal participant in the activity. In his flashback to the abuse when he was 6 years old, "*I am in the bathroom with my grandfather. I am naked and he is pressing me against the radiator on the wall. I remember the sensation of the back of my head touching the top of the radiator* [which gives an idea how tall he was at the age of six] *but I see my grandfather and myself as from the outside. In this picture, I am 38 and bald and my grandfather is very frail*". (In reality his grandfather was 55 and fit and well, at the time of the abuse.)

The patient was asked to comment on this gross visual distortion. He realised that he had always updated the flashback throughout his life to make him seem as adult as he could be. He and the therapist worked on the meaning of this updating.

As he seemed more adult and stronger than the abuser it seemed to mean: "It was my fault". Once he realised the link between the visual cognitive distortion and the meaning, he was able to change the image to a more realistic one. He made the image of himself into a small boy and his grandfather went back to being 55. He looked at the new image in session and would transform the old image to the new one, if the old one came back. He then said to the therapist, in wonder: "How could it have been my fault, I was only 6 years old."

The more realistic image allowed this patient to realise in a fundamental way that his guilt and recrimination were misplaced. His symptoms improved and at the end of treatment he was able to start work. In effect his goal system underwent a major change from being one involving distorted imagery of being trapped in abuse for which he was responsible to accepting himself as a victim. Recognition that he was victimised, represented in the form of the more realistic visual mental image, allowed development to recommence.

CONCLUSION

Traumatic memories and the images derived from them have powerful effects upon the self. Here we have argued that this might occur because images are derived from goals. One function of an image might be to maintain a set of dysfunctional beliefs that in turn preserve the goal system and protect it from the need for change. Another aspect of images is that they may be derived from different types of goals. Those deriving from goals that function to reduce discrepancies do not intrude into consciousness and hijack attention. In contrast, images derived from goals that increase discrepancy unless constrained by discrepancy-reducing goals are effectively out of control and when activated intrude into consciousness and hijack attention. Linking such goals to images associated with constraining goals appears to reduce psychopathological feelings and thoughts. Possibly this occurs because images that imply a constraining goal, in some sense bring about the implementation of that goal in the working self. Perhaps it is this supposed goal change that underlies the claim by many survivors of trauma that they are now a different self from the self that existed prior to their traumatic experience.

REFERENCES

Carver, C. S., & Scheier, M. F. (1982). Control theory: A useful conceptual framework for personality-social, clinical, and health psychology. *Psychological Bulletin*, *92*, 111–135.

Carver, C. S., & Scheier, M. F. (1998). *On the self-regulation of behavior.* New York: Cambridge University Press.

Carver, C. S., & Scheier, M. F. (1999). Themes and issues in the self-regulation of behavior. In R. S. Wyer Jr. (Ed.), *Advances in social cognition* (Vol. 12). Mahwah, NJ: Lawrence Erlbaum Associates Inc.

Conway, M. A. (2001). Sensory perceptual episodic memory and its context: autobiographical memory. *Philosophical Transactions of the Royal Society, London, B*, *356*(1413), 1375–1384.

Conway, M. A., & Pleydell-Pearce, C. W. (2000) The construction of autobiographical memories in the self memory system. *Psychological Review*, *107*, 261–288.

Conway, M. A., Singer, J. A., & Tagini, A. (2004). The self and autobiographical memory: Correspondence and coherence. *Social Cognition.*

Dadds, M. R., Bovbjerg, D., Redd, W. H., & Cutmore, T. (1997). Imagery and human classical conditioning. *Psychological Bulletin*, *121*, 89–103.

Dadds, M. R., Hawes, D., Schaefer, B., & Vaka, K. (2004). Individual differences and reports of aversions. *Memory*, *12*, 462–466.

Day, S. J., Holmes, E. A., & Hackmann, E. (2004). Occurrence of imagery and its link with early memories in agoraphobia. *Memory*, *12*, 416–427.

Ehlers, A., & Clark, D. M. (2000). A cognitive model of posttraumatic stress disorder. *Behaviour Research and Therapy*, *38*, 319–345.

Ehlers, A., Hackmann, A., & Michael, T. (2004). Intrusive re-experiencing in post-traumatic stress disorder: Phenomenology, theory, and therapy. *Memory*, *12*, 403–415.

Gilbert, P., & Irons, C. (2004). A pilot exploration of the use of compassionate images in a group of self-critical people. *Memory*, *12*, 507–516.

Grey, N., Young, K., & Holmes, E. (2002). Cognitive restructuring within reliving: A treatment for peritraumatic emotional "hotspots" in posttraumatic stress disorder. *Behavioural and Cognitive Psychotherapy*, *30*, 37–56.

Hirsch, C. R., Meynen, T., & Clark, D. M. (2004). Negative self-imagery in social anxiety contaminates social interactions. *Memory*, *12*, 496–506.

Holmes, E. A., Grey, N., & Young, K. A. D. (in press). Intrusive images and "hotspots" of trauma memories in posttraumatic stress disorder: An exploratory investigation of emotions and cognitive themes. *Journal of Behavior Therapy and Experimental Psychiatry.*

Horowitz, M., Wilner, N., & Alvarez, W. (1979) Impact of Events Scale: A measure of subjective stress. *Psychosomatic Medicine*, *41*(3), 209–218.

Mansell, W., & Lam, D. (2004). A preliminary study of autobiographical memory in remitted bipolar and unipolar depression and the role of imagery in the specificity of memory. *Memory*, *12*, 437–446.

May, J., Andrade, J., Panabokke, N., & Kavanagh, D. (2004). Images of desire: Cognitive models of craving. *Memory, 12,* 447–461.

Morrison, A. P. (2004). The use of imagery in cognitive therapy for psychosis: A case example. *Memory, 12,* 517–524.

Oatley, K. (1992). *The best laid schemes. The psychology of emotions.* Cambridge: Cambridge University Press.

Osman, S., Cooper, M., Hackmann, A., & Veale, D. (2004). Spontaneously accurring images and early memories in people with body dysmorphic disorder. *Memory, 12,* 428–436.

Tulving, E. (1983). *Elements of episodic memory.* Oxford: Clarendon Press.

Subject Index

For Product Safety Concerns and Information please contact our EU representative GPSR@taylorandfrancis.com Taylor & Francis Verlag GmbH, Kaufingerstraße 24, 80331 München, Germany

T - #0198 - 270225 - C0 - 272/202/9 - PB - 9781841699677 - Gloss Lamination